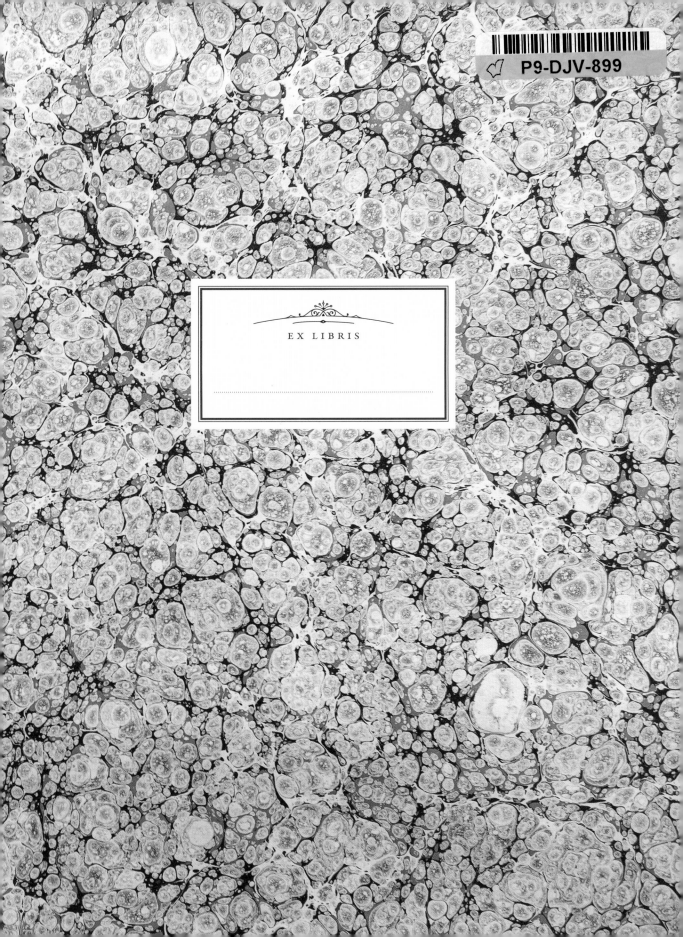

EX LIBRIS

THE
GENTLEMAN'S
GUIDE
TO
GROOMING

....

The Quintessential Handbook
for the Modern Man

C<small>APT</small>. P<small>EABODY</small> F<small>AWCETT</small>, <small>RET</small>.

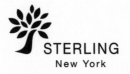

STERLING
New York

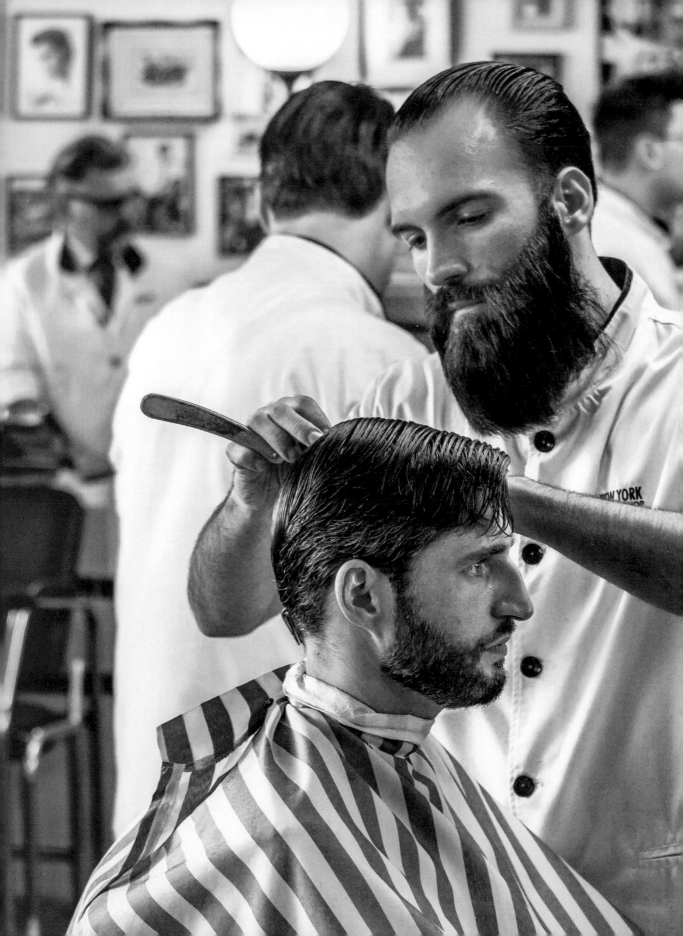

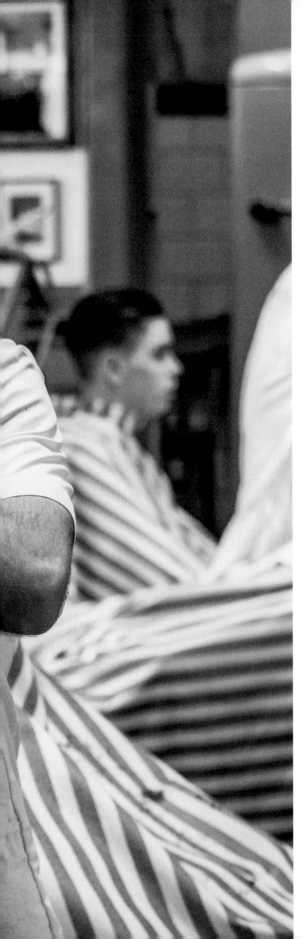

The Captain should like to take this opportunity to thank
Gordon, Iain, Allie, Cate, & Lily, without whom this book
would not have been possible.

All Hail the Hirsute!

STERLING
New York

An Imprint of Sterling Publishing, Co., Inc.
1166 Avenue of the Americas
New York, NY 10016

Text © 2017 by Captain Fawcett Limited
Commissioned photography © 2017 by Captain Fawcett Limited
and Jacqui Small, an imprint of the Quarto Group

ISBN 978-1-4549-2240-7

Distributed in Canada by Sterling Publishing Co., Inc.
c/o Canadian Manda Group, 664 Annette Street
Toronto, Ontario, M6S 2C8, Canada

For information about custom editions, special sales,
and premium and corporate purchases, please contact
Sterling Special Sales at 800-805-5489 or specialsales@
sterlingpublishing.com.

Manufactured in China

2 4 6 8 10 9 7 5 3 1

sterlingpublishing.com

A complete list of image credits appears on page 176.

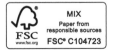

MIX
Paper from
responsible sources
FSC® C104723

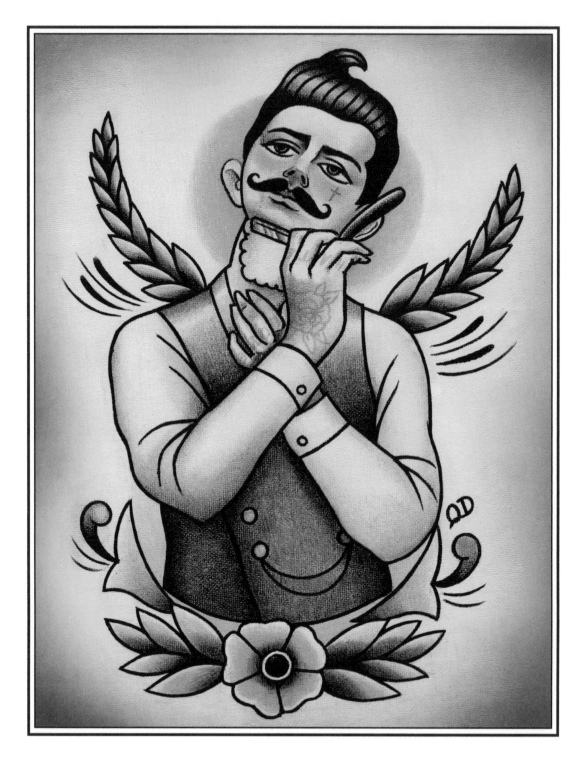

The distinctive and inimitable style of Queyn Dinh's Tattoo Flash as fine art can be seen on the walls and arms of many a good barber.

THE
CONTENTS

INTRODUCTION

M Y DEAR CHUMS, how refreshing to see your refined noses in a good book! To those readers who have yet to make my acquaintance, allow me to introduce myself. I am Captain Peabody Fawcett, Royal Navy, Retired, purveyor and manufacturer of simply first-class gentleman's grooming requisites, intrepid world traveler, and adventurer to boot.

As a long-time connoisseur of hair in all its glorious manifestations, I was delighted to receive an invitation to compile *The Gentleman's Guide to Grooming*. To muster this history and modern gentleman's guide, I have journeyed far and wide, encountering astounding characters and follicular experts whose generosity sharing work and stories is without parallel. Their contributions are illustrated by images from some of the world's best photographers, unmistakable artists every one of them. I have been enlightened and entertained, and I am most sincerely grateful to them all.

I hold in high regard those invisible qualities of courage, honor, and service that reside in the hearts of gallant gentlemen yet well understand that how one presents oneself to the world is of paramount importance. How a fellow chooses to frame his face is the mark of a man, and it has a bearing on how he will be judged by society. The long and the short of it is that hair matters. From the first flourish of facial follicles heralding the beginning of manhood, at some juncture every chap must decide how best to polish and present himself, whether to blend in or stand out. Fashion, faith, class, culture, and profession all shape one's beard or indeed the shaving of it, and to be well-groomed has a profound influence on a chap's confidence and self-esteem. A considered appearance allows one to put one's best foot forward and maintain a stiff upper lip, regardless.

Rajah or revolutionary, soldier or schoolboy, every man from poor prisoner to glittering prince has at some time had a haircut or shave. His barber might be lavish with hot towels in a scented city salon or own little more than a broken mirror on a Kolkata street corner, but a gentleman's impulse to pay attention to his appearance has been the same throughout history. Whether ascetic monk renouncing vanity or dapper man about town fully embracing it, by styling his hair a particular way a gentleman projects something of his personality, social standing, and sense of wellbeing.

Join me as I celebrate adventurous gentlemen everywhere—and some most memorable ladies—from all walks of life and as I stroll through time and travel around the world. Onward chaps!

All Hail the Hirsute!

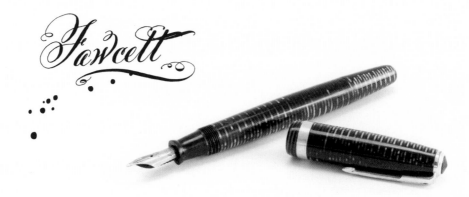

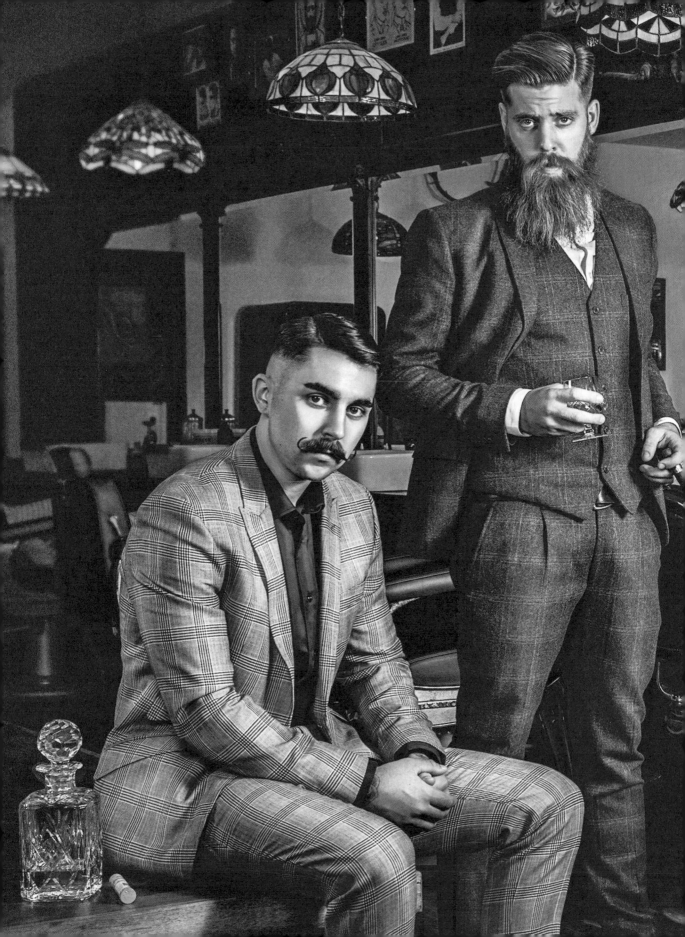

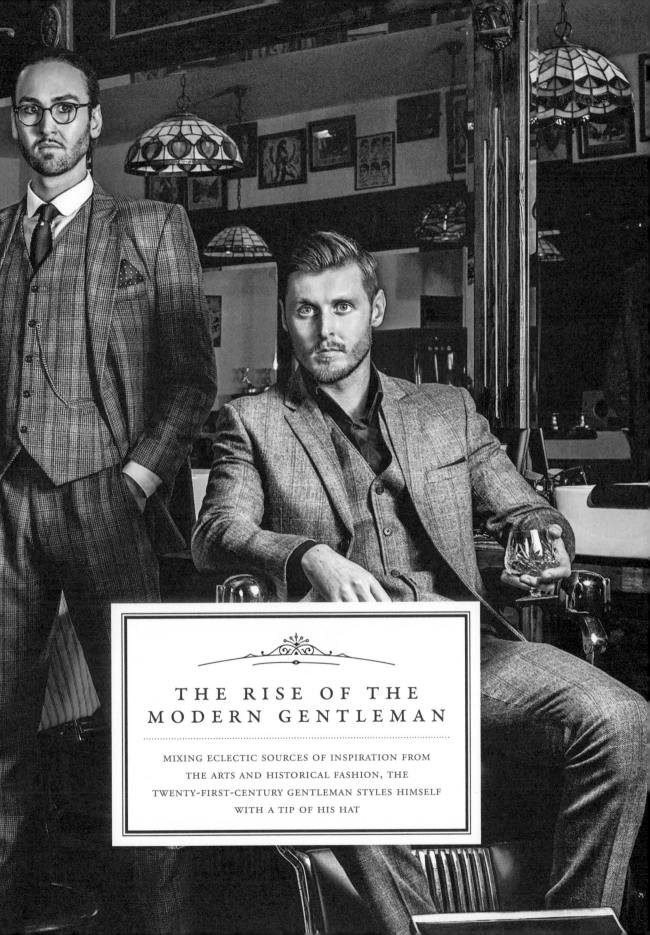

THE RISE OF THE
MODERN GENTLEMAN

MIXING ECLECTIC SOURCES OF INSPIRATION FROM
THE ARTS AND HISTORICAL FASHION, THE
TWENTY-FIRST-CENTURY GENTLEMAN STYLES HIMSELF
WITH A TIP OF HIS HAT

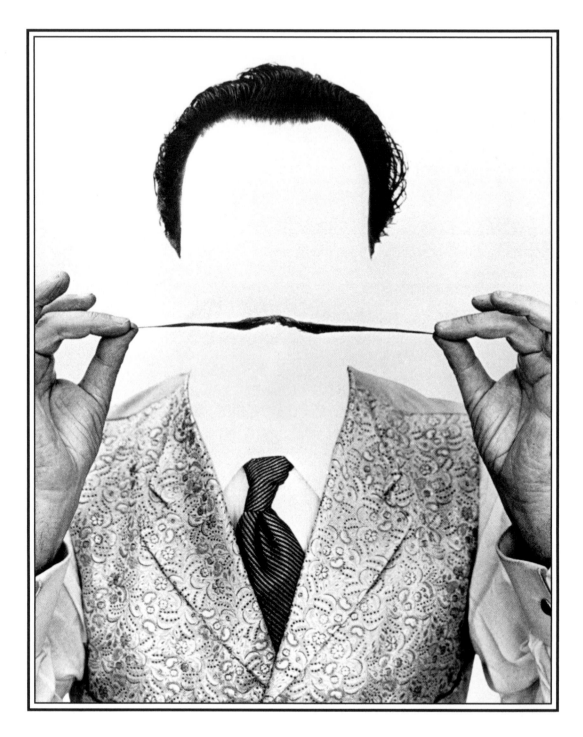

Who is the modern gentleman?

I CONFESS TO being an inquisitive cove, well acquainted with fellows from all cuts of jib and strata of society. I count myself as fortunate since there is nothing as delightful as the company of a roguish gentleman, or, for that matter, a gentlemanly rogue. Allow me to share with you tales of varying height and to present characters as colorful and manifold as whiskers on a well-groomed chin.

T HE MODERN GENTLEMAN'S reputation is tribute to a way of life that gives expression to the highest personal standards. In the twenty-first century, to be a gentleman is no longer an accident of birth but a conscious decision, the decision to choose affability over surliness, discipline over disorder, and consideration over churlishness. The true gentleman is a steadfast figure, enduring through history, transcending culture and class, and always adapting to his time. In its current manifestation, released from a code of etiquette as suffocating as a starched collar on a summer afternoon, to be a modern gentleman is to present a distinctive personality defined by healthy self-esteem and the ability to make the best of one's given assets in every walk of life.

In yesteryear, the social life of a gentleman revolved around an archaic code of conduct, the rigid observation of which was essential to avoid tripping into faux pas and facing ridicule. The world of the modern gentleman is far more relaxed and free from snooty constraint: he is able to celebrate his individuality with distinctive personal flair. While appreciating that manners still matter, today's gentlemen understand that many social cues are nonverbal, so one's appearance has lasting influence. The gentleman's desire to make a positive impression by virtue of his good grooming is due not to narcissism nor purely in the interests of self-advancement, rather that he knows scruffiness is as distracting as over-preening and wishes to direct attention to his character and conversation.

In modern grooming there are no firm rules but fundamental values focusing on health and hygiene, and these values tend not to be prohibitive but instead invite today's gentleman to be mindful of diverse routines and rituals and give him the liberty to make them his own. The modern gentleman enjoys the time dedicated to grooming, whether it's banter with the barber during a hot-towel shave, relaxing in a bath scented with oils, or a quick manicure before a meeting. As essential to health as good diet and adequate exercise, time to oneself is never wasted but is a vital part of maintaining wellbeing and a buoyant demeanor. In matters of style, whether to wear a beard, mustache,

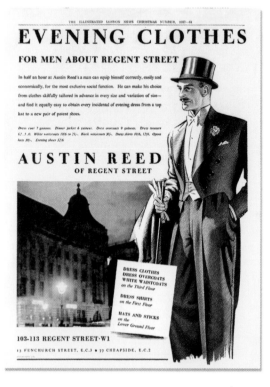

or sport a close shave is usually the decision of the individual, as few walks of modern life insist on severely restrictive beard or hair styles.

An unkempt, slovenly presentation suggests lack of self-awareness, laziness, or low state of mind, which at worst is offensive to one's acquaintances and at best flags justified cause for concern in friends. It is well documented that improved appearance is a great boost to a fellow's mood and sprucing up enables even a shy chap to step into a room with élan. At the other end of the grooming spectrum, excessive vanity is not the mark of a real gentleman, who is known for the attention he gives to others, not for how much he devotes to himself.

In his sixteenth-century guide to courtly etiquette, *Il Cortegiano*, Baldassare Castiglione writes about *"sprezzatura,"* an

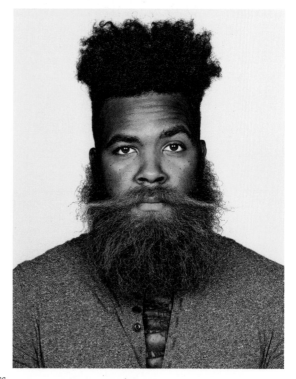

artfully studied nonchalance belying the effort necessary to acquire a variety of skills, from swordsmanship and dancing to writing poetry and playing music. The modern gentleman has much in common with his Renaissance brother; after all, a man who wears his accomplishments lightly is perennially attractive. We no longer presume the gentleman must be born to nobility—social adaptability and the ability to put any company at ease is much prized in the world of the modern gentleman, and snobbery no longer has a place. He need not be conventionally handsome, either. What matters is being authentic to one's personal style, paying attention to detail, whether in tailoring, skincare, or behavior, and, above all, being comfortable in one's own skin.

Respectful of tradition but not restricted by it, there is nothing old-fashioned about the gentleman of today. Renewing his style to keep pace with the times, he is flexible and resilient, with unimpeachable principles and a warm wit. In an uncertain world of increasingly abrupt change, where public life often seems overshadowed by bad news and belligerence, he sets an enduring standard of personal integrity and honor. Gracious, groomed, and good natured, the modern gentleman is an urbane role model for our times, as indeed he ever was.

An Age Apart
Brandon Baker displays the quiet confidence of a well-dressed man (above). 1930s advertisement for Austin Reed's flagship store in Regent Street, London, which opened in 1911 and offered the elegance one might require for a night on the town (opposite). ❧

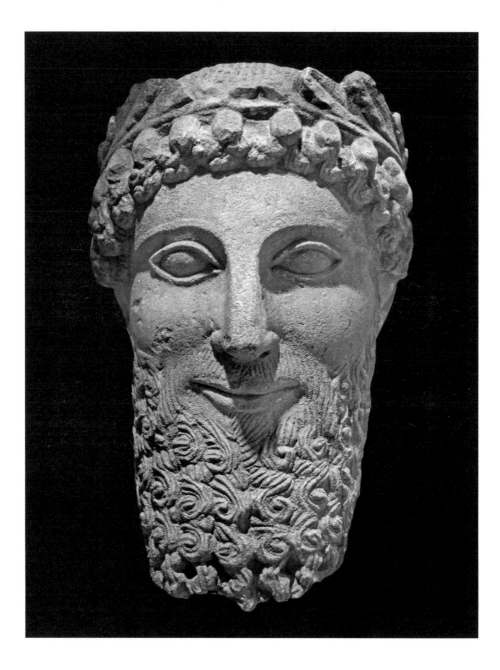

GENTLEMANLY ORIGINS

History exerts a powerful influence. The foppish fads and fashions of the past, be it pirate or prince, soldier or shaman, desperado or dandy, echo in the modern gentleman's wardrobe. As ever, one's style speaks volumes.

A Walk through Time

FACIAL HAIR IN bushy splendor is all the rage at the moment. Indeed, hirsute is hip. But the story of men's appearance over the millennia is a complex one, hair on the head and face having come and gone according to the whims of kings and clergymen, in line with the tide of fashion or simply for the sake of looking good. Hair has been worn long, short, shorn, dyed, powdered, and curled; and beards, mustaches, and sideburns have been carefully cultivated at times and strictly suppressed at others. The beard has been subject to religious pronouncements, health advisory warnings, cod theories, and even fiscal necessity—eighteenth-century Russian csar Peter the Great levied a tax on what the *Moby-Dick* writer Herman Melville once described as the "suburbs of the chin."

Of course, man has long enjoyed the possibility of the beard since time immemorial; it provided protection for prehistoric hominids against cold, wind, and sun. But sometime before 2000BC came the notion of shaving. Given that the depilatory implements would have been fairly primitive, it must have been a painful and bloody business. Flint was used, for example, and, in Polynesia, seashells.

The pre-eminent figures of the early tribes were medicine men who also served as barbers. These societies believed that good and bad spirits entered the body through the hairs on the head and the only way to drive them out was to cut the hair. The Ancient Egyptians were superstitious

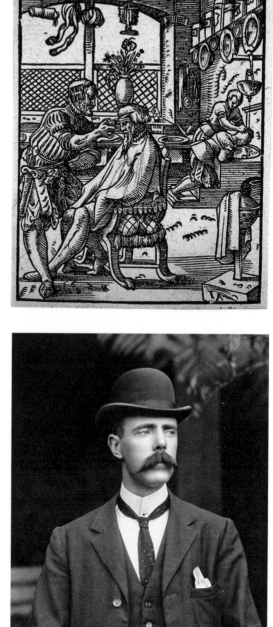

Beard, Barber, and Bowler
Luxuriant, curled beards were the rage in Ancient Greece (opposite). A medieval barber shearing a fetching fringe (above right). Bowler hat, starched collar, handkerchief, watch chain, and smartly groomed mustache: de rigueur for a day at the office c.1900 (right). ✳

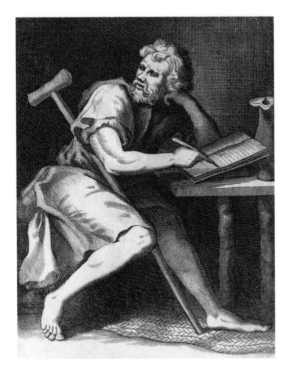

about hair, and priests shaved their entire bodies every few days. We are familiar, of course, with the beards of the pharaohs. These were often fake, hooked over the ears. Even the Eigthteenth Dynasty female pharaoh, Hatshepsut, wore a fake beard to emphasize her authority.

The Ancient Greeks, forever pondering the nature of being, believed that hair—especially the beard—was an indicator of male superiority, but Alexander the Great put an end to that notion by shaving. The 22-year-old emperor was keen for people to identify him with the youthful, smooth-chinned paragons of health and beauty that classical sculptors depicted in the representation of Greece's heroic age. Having previously sported luxuriant beards, Greek men began to follow Alexander's example and shave. Thus, the barbershop become a feature on any fashionable Ancient Greek

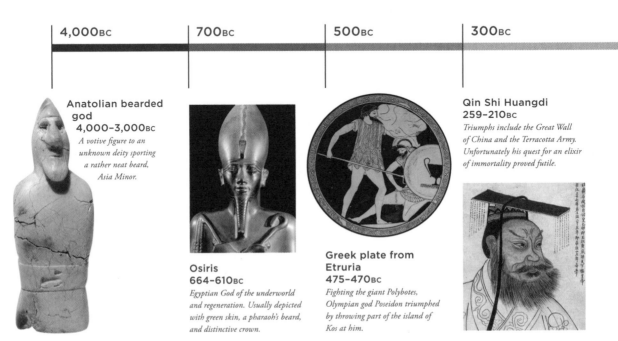

4,000BC   **700**BC   **500**BC   **300**BC

Anatolian bearded god
4,000–3,000BC
A votive figure to an unknown deity sporting a rather neat beard, Asia Minor.

Osiris
664–610BC
Egyptian God of the underworld and regeneration. Usually depicted with green skin, a pharaoh's beard, and distinctive crown.

Greek plate from Etruria
475–470BC
Fighting the giant Polybotes, Olympian god Poseidon triumphed by throwing part of the island of Kos at him.

Qin Shi Huangdi
259–210BC
Triumphs include the Great Wall of China and the Terracotta Army. Unfortunately his quest for an elixir of immortality proved futile.

street. The Romans, too, enjoyed the services of barbers; an individual named Ticinius Mena first introduced them from Sicily in 296BC. The barber's became a place for exchanging gossip and whiling away an afternoon.

In the Middle Ages, barbers became jacks of all trades: pulling teeth, dressing wounds, and performing operations as well as cutting hair and shaving. The first trade organization was formed in France in 1096, after the archbishop of Rouen banned the wearing of beards. In 1308, the Worshipful Company of Barbers was instituted in London, but barbers and surgeons went their separate ways in the eigthteenth century.

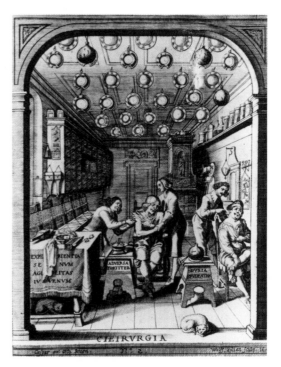

Philosophers and Physicians
Epictetus, Greek stoic (opposite). Interior of a barber-surgeon's establishment: two men receiving minor surgical treatment, showing bloodletting basins and jars of leeches hanging from the ceiling c. 1652 (right). ❧

| 100BC | 100BC | AD600 | 1100 |

Alexander mosaic from the House of the Faun, Pompeii (detail)
c.100BC
Darius III of Persia battling Alexander the Great. He was eventually killed by traitors from his own army.

Svetovid, four-headed god
c.150–1BC
Slavic god depicted on the silver Gundestrup cauldron embodying war, fertility, and divination. His accoutrements include a sword and a drinking horn.

Sutton Hoo helmet
EARLY SEVENTH CENTURY
Engraved with fine facial hair, this is one of only four known complete helmets from Anglo-Saxon England.

Lewis chess piece
1150–1200
These handsomely bearded Scandinavian walrus ivory chess pieces often have expressions that are decidedly comical to modern eyes.

Until the eigthteenth century, barber-surgeons' duties included de-lousing, primitive dentistry, lancing abscesses, setting bone fractures, and bloodletting. To advertise this latter service, bowls of blood would often be displayed in the windows of their shops, and, when that was ruled to be unhygienic, the barber's pole was adopted. It signified the rod that customers clasped to make their veins bulge for ease of bloodletting. The red-and-white stripes symbolized the resulting blood-soaked bandages, and the gold orb at the top represented the basin used to collect the blood. Delightful.

The second half of the eigthteenth century brought great change to the profession of barber. Suddenly, powdered wigs became the height of fashion, driven, as was often the case, by royal taste. King Louis XIII of France wore a wig to disguise his bald pate in 1624, and the habit began to spread. Shoulder-length wigs became de rigueur at the English royal court following the restoration of Charles II to the throne in 1660, so barbers also became wig-makers and enhanced their income with wig-maintenance. In the eigthteenth century, men began to powder their wigs, giving them a distinctive off-white color while, from about 1770 onward, women sported fantastic, towering wigs that boasted every color of the rainbow. The age of the wig was effectively brought to an end in Britain in 1795, when the government introduced a tax on hair powder of one guinea a year.

Get cracking!
Britain's finest hour: preparing for heroic action at a Royal Airforce Fighter Station in 1942. ❦

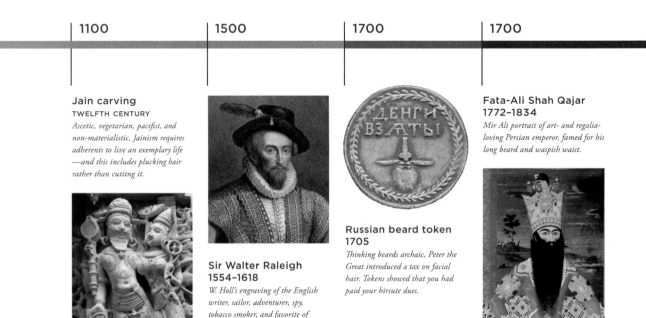

1100

Jain carving
TWELFTH CENTURY
Ascetic, vegetarian, pacifist, and non-materialistic, Jainism requires adherents to live an exemplary life —and this includes plucking hair rather than cutitng it.

1500

Sir Walter Raleigh
1554–1618
W. Holl's engraving of the English writer, sailor, adventurer, spy, tobacco smoker, and favorite of Queen Elizabeth I.

1700

Russian beard token
1705
Thinking beards archaic, Peter the Great introduced a tax on facial hair. Tokens showed that you had paid your hirsute dues.

1700

Fata-Ali Shah Qajar
1772–1834
Mir Ali portrait of art- and regalia-loving Persian emperor, famed for his long beard and waspish waist.

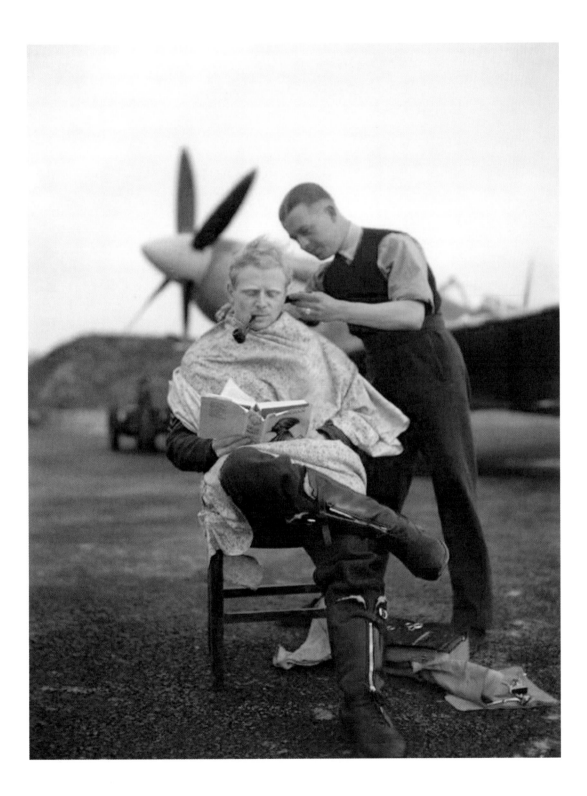

The nineteenth century was *the* time for facial hair. Beards, mutton-chops, luxuriant Piccadilly weepers, and bulging sideburns graced the visages of men imitating the styles worn by heroes returning from the Crimea. Grooming products, too, grew in popularity. Doctors, meanwhile, prescribed the growth of beards as a means of warding off illness, the beard serving as a filter that would capture impurities before they were inhaled. The Victorian notion of masculinity, the male as patriarch, was reinforced by a full beard, distinguishing husband very clearly from wife.

An invention by American businessman King Camp Gillette killed off the beard for 60 years or more. His safety razor caught on and men were once again becoming increasingly clean-shaven as the twentieth century dawned.

The exception was the British military. After the Crimean War mustaches were made compulsory for serving soldiers, a regulation abolished only in October 1916, by which time men too young to grow much facial hair were being recruited. Nonetheless, many soldiers continued to sport mustaches.

Only movie stars and mustache-twirling villains were hirsute above the top lip as the twenties segued into the thirties, and Adolph Hitler's toothbrush mustache understandably made men reluctant to celebrate facial hair after World War II. But a generation growing up in the swinging 1960s embraced hair in every shape or form, and long hair and beards curled down onto smocks and kaftans. In the seventies, sideburns sprouted, but in the era of Thatcher and Reagan we were once again clean-shaven.

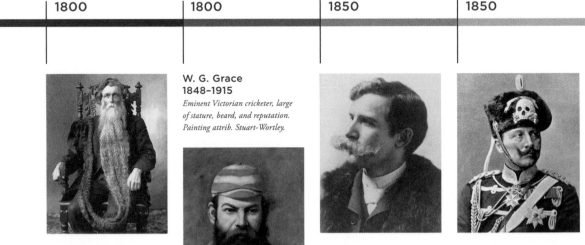

1800   1800   1850   1850

**Hans Langseth
1846–1927**
The longest beard in history—over 17 feet. On Langseth's death it was donated to the Smithsonian Institute.

**W. G. Grace
1848–1915**
Eminent Victorian cricketer, large of stature, beard, and reputation. Painting attrib. Stuart-Wortley.

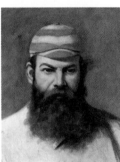

**Henry Wellcome
1853–1936**
Flamboyant pharmaceutical entrepreneur and philanthropist who founded The Wellcome Trust.

**Kaiser Wilhelm II
1859–1941**
Bombastic and bright with an excellent taste in mustaches and hats but unfortunately bellicose.

In the latter decades of the twentieth century, as society became more accepting, openly gay men championed luxuriant mustaches and, on occasion, bushy beards.

Millennial men have shown themselves to be no upholders of the old mores regarding facial hair and beards, as such exponents of hirsute pride can be seen most everywhere. A group of British men formed the Beard Liberation Front in 1995, and five years later they protested by waggling their beards at "clean-shaven capitalism." Now there are beard competitions and beard movements around the world, including the World Beard Championship, and the business of maintaining beards and mustaches has gone through the roof.

It would appear that the "suburbs of the chin" will remain occupied for some time to come.

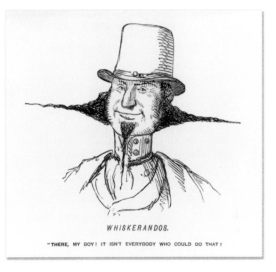

WHISKERANDOS.

"THERE, MY BOY! IT ISN'T EVERYBODY WHO COULD DO THAT!"

Winning by a Whisker
Beard competitions are nothing new. An early whisker-wearer lampooned by caricaturist John Leech. ✻

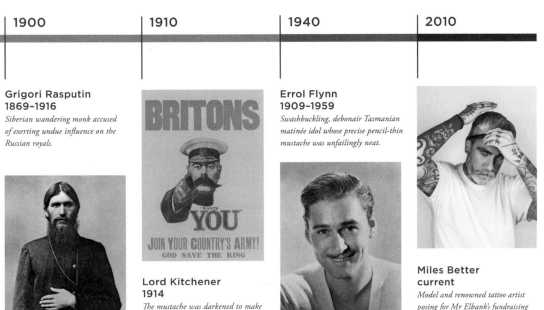

1900

1910

1940

2010

Grigori Rasputin
1869–1916
Siberian wandering monk accused of exerting undue influence on the Russian royals.

Lord Kitchener
1914
The mustache was darkened to make Kitchener appear extra commanding.

Errol Flynn
1909–1959
Swashbuckling, debonair Tasmanian matinée idol whose precise pencil-thin mustache was unfailingly neat.

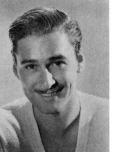

Miles Better
current
Model and renowned tattoo artist posing for Mr Elbank's fundraising #Project60 pack of playing cards.

Religious Traditions

HAIR AND RELIGION have gone strand in strand since the days when shamans cast out demons by cutting hair. Hair can signify purity, spirituality, a oneness with God, and a respect for the perfection of God's creation. Why mess around with perfection?

For a Sikh, keeping one's natural hair uncut and covered is a mark of respect for the will of God, and it is so significant that the practice has a name: Kesh. Turbans function as symbols of faith, practical headwear, and, for modern Sikh gentlemen, a stylish way to add a dash of color to a sober city suit. Hindus, in contrast, have many rituals involving shaving their heads. It begins at the age of four when Hindu children—girls and boys—have their heads shaved in a ritual known as Chudakarana Samskara. Hair is perceived as an adornment. Therefore, by shaving the hair, the child is forced to learn humility and devotion. This is carried through to adulthood: at the Kumbh Mela—the mass Hindu pilgrimage during which tens of thousands gather to bathe in a sacred river—the first ritual that most of the pilgrims perform is the Mundana, the shaving of the head.

When the young Prince Siddhartha left the comfort and luxury of his palace to seek enlightenment and become the Buddha, one of the first things he did was to shave his head. Buddhist monks, therefore, completely shave their hair and beards as a sign of their commitment to the holy life and as an act of renunciation of the striving for beauty. A Buddhist monk will shave at least once every two weeks or if hair grows beyond a length of two finger breadths. He is not allowed to dye or pluck out gray hairs, as they serve as reminders of old age and the impermanence of everything, a concept important to Buddhists.

But many other religions revere hair. The Amish view hair—the hair on men's chins in particular—as sacrosanct. They grow a beard but, interestingly, never wear a mustache, a practice dating back to when soldiers always wore them and the peaceable Amish were keen to dissociate themselves with violence. In fact, cutting an Amish man's beard against his will is now regarded as a hate crime.

Rastafarians never cut their hair or, indeed, brush it. They follow the strictures of Leviticus 21:5: "They shall not make baldness upon their head, neither shall they shave off the corner of their beard, nor make any cuttings in their flesh." Male Hassidic Jews grow their sideburns—known as peyos—and they can be curled or tucked behind the ears. The Torah—the first five books of the Hebrew scriptures—forbids the destruction or shaving of the hairs.

Men of Good Faith
Top row left to right: Hindu sadhu (India), Greek Orthodox priest (Greece), Sikh man (India), Hassidic Jew (Israel). Bottom row left to right: Buddhist monk (Myanmar), Rastafarian (Jamaica), Tao monk (China), Amish man (Pennsylvania). 🕮

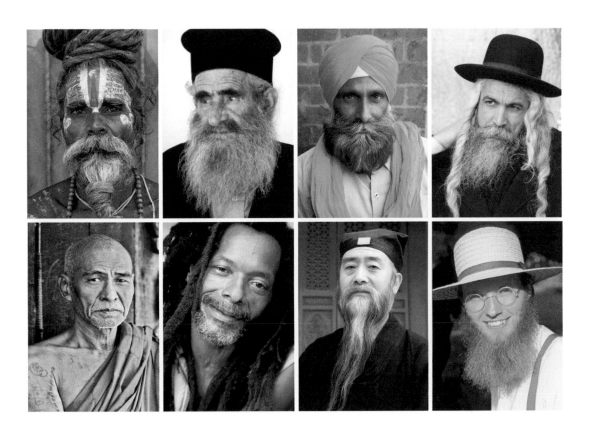

The Quran does not prescribe the wearing of beards, but the Hadith (the collected sayings of the prophet Muhammad) contains a passage ordering followers to grow beards. Therefore, some Muslims believe that a beard is an absolute requirement for a man of faith. Both men and women are required to remove armpit and pubic hair at least every forty days.

Christianity's relationship with facial hair has been tricky. For St. Augustine, beards were good: "The beard signifies the courageous; the beard distinguishes the grown men, the active, the vigorous." But after him began regular—and fairly random—beard bans by religious figures, including Wolfsan, archbishop of York, in 1023. The twelfth-century bishop of Rouen excommunicated all who failed to shave. When some men hung on to their beards, they were beaten, and rioting broke out. The situation became so dangerous that King Louis VII of France shaved his beard in solidarity with the clergy. Smooth chins then became fashionable at court, a fashion that, to the bishop's relief, spread among the populace.

For some, hirsuteness is the next thing to godliness; others see it as a symbol of earthly adornment that must be removed. But hair, as we can see, remains a powerful symbol for many religions.

Rules & Regulations

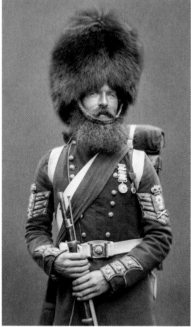

HAIR MEANS A great deal to a man. A well-styled head of hair and a neatly trimmed beard can make him feel chipper, raise his self-esteem, and give him the wherewithal to take on the challenges the world poses for him. Therefore, to force a man to cut off his hair and his beard destroys what often makes him an autonomous, distinct individual. It is also designed to reinforce submissiveness and obedience. This has been employed in countless situations in history, whether in the case of defeated troops being forced to cut their hair and shave or a convict being whipped into shape by a disciplinarian governor. The warlike Spartans punished men perceived to be cowards by shaving off half their beards, exposing them to public humiliation and mockery. Roman officials routinely shaved the heads of persecuted early Christians to humiliate them and subject them to ridicule.

Convicts have been subjected to having their identities expunged through being shorn. Prison authorities claim that prisoners' hair is cut for reasons of cleanliness and hygiene, to prevent infestation or infection, or even, somewhat ridiculously, to prevent drains being clogged. The enforced shearing of hair is, of course, common in the military around the world. Commanders aspire to create a unit that thinks and acts as one, that is willing to sacrifice itself for the good of the whole. But once it was different; it made sense for men to sport fearsome facial hair as they went into battle to inspire terror in an enemy who equated such a display of wild hair with brutishness. However, we know that Vikings carried combs and tweezers, ensuring they were handsomely groomed during a day of plundering and pillaging. British soldiers were ordered to grow facial hair in their wars in India and Asia to impress cultures who respected or feared facial hair. In the mid-nineteenth century, facial hair was encouraged for another reason: the bitter cold of a Crimean winter persuaded officers to encourage all ranks to grow beards, mustaches,

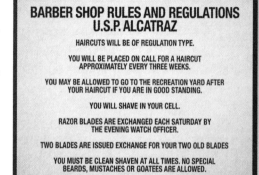

BARBER SHOP RULES AND REGULATIONS U.S.P. ALCATRAZ

HAIRCUTS WILL BE OF REGULATION TYPE.

YOU WILL BE PLACED ON CALL FOR A HAIRCUT APPROXIMATELY EVERY THREE WEEKS.

YOU MAY BE ALLOWED TO GO TO THE RECREATION YARD AFTER YOUR HAIRCUT IF YOU ARE IN GOOD STANDING.

YOU WILL SHAVE IN YOUR CELL.

RAZOR BLADES ARE EXCHANGED EACH SATURDAY BY THE EVENING WATCH OFFICER.

TWO BLADES ARE ISSUED EXCHANGE FOR YOUR TWO OLD BLADES

YOU MUST BE CLEAN SHAVEN AT ALL TIMES. NO SPECIAL BEARDS, MUSTACHES OR GOATEES ARE ALLOWED.

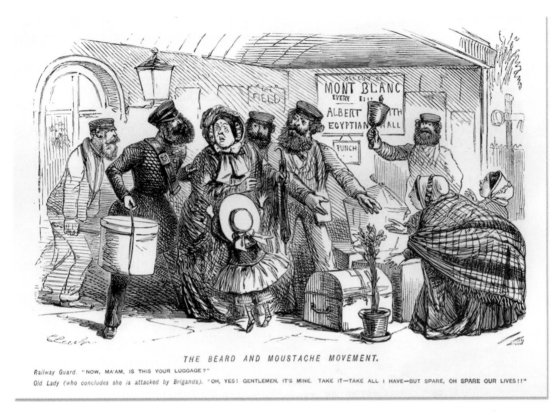

THE BEARD AND MOUSTACHE MOVEMENT.

Railway Guard. "NOW, MA'AM, IS THIS YOUR LUGGAGE?"
Old Lady (who concludes she is attacked by Brigands). "OH, YES! GENTLEMEN, IT'S MINE. TAKE IT—TAKE ALL I HAVE—BUT SPARE, OH SPARE OUR LIVES!!"

and side-whiskers to combat frostbite. Hirsute soldiers returning from the war led to the last great period when facial hair achieved widespread popularity. Men wanted to identify with the valiant troops, and this led to a series of cartoons in *Punch* magazine satirizing what it called "The Beard and Moustache Movement." After that, regulations were introduced that prevented soldiers from shaving above the top lip, an edict that remained in place until October 1916 when Lieutenant-General Sir Nevil Macready, who apparently detested his own mustache, issued an order abolishing that regulation and promptly removed his own.

French soldiers had been permitted to wear full beards from the Napoleonic era, although the tradition gradually faded from the start of the twentieth century. This did not stop World War I French soldiers being nicknamed *poilus* (hairy ones) because of their facial hair. A regulation of 1975 banned French military personnel from growing a beard or mustache unless they were out of uniform. Now, only the sappers of the French Foreign Legion are allowed to wear beards. Meanwhile, in the United States Army, Air Force, and Marine Corps, beards are banned unless there are religious reasons for growing one.

Ruled by the Head
Beard and bearskin provide ample insulation (above left). Facial hair was banned in the notorious San Francisco jail (bottom left). Punch cartoon poking fun at those who feared the beard (top). ❧

Myths & Fairytales

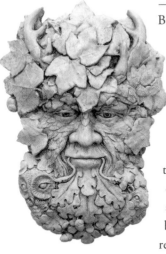

BEFORE AROUND 500BC, mythic heroes and gods were depicted by classical Greek artists as resembling Greek warriors of the time. They wore tunics or military clothing, their hair was long, and they sported abundant beards; all, that is, except poor Apollo, who was condemned to eternal, beardless, fresh-faced youth. By the end of the fifth century, however, portrayals of heroes and gods show them having shed their armor and tunics and shaved their beards. Only Zeus and Poseidon, two of the more senior members of the divine pantheon, remained hirsute, probably to dignify them with an air of age, wisdom, and authority. Achilles, hero of *The Iliad*, Homer's epic poem of the Trojan War, was always shown as a beautiful, beardless young man, but that may have simply been borrowed from the poem's description of him. It may, however, also have reflected the homoerotic predilections of the Athenian elite of the time. Ultimately, however, the truth is probably that the depiction of facial hair was doomed because beauty and youth had become conflated with immortality in the art of classical Greece.

A white beard features in one of the greatest hits of the Middle Ages—the eleventh–twelfth century *Song of Roland*, an epic poem based on the 778 Battle of Roncevaux. In the poem, written some 300 years after the death of Charlemagne, the great king's most significant attribute is his large white beard. As the poem describes it: "His beard is white and his head is hoary." In fact, Charlemagne's appearance, especially his beard, is a leitmotif used throughout the work. The reality was, however, that in Charlemagne's day the Franks over whom he ruled wore their hair cropped and their beards clipped. Charlemagne is furnished with a luxuriant beard in the poem to endow him with a mythical authority and wisdom.

Vikings are often depicted as unkempt, violent warriors, but the truth about this marauding people who colonized large parts of Europe between the eighth and the eleventh centuries was actually very different.

Legendary Beards
The Green Man, age-old English woodland spirit (above). Every child's favorite, St. Nicholas AKA Santa Claus (right). Another terrifying feather in Bluebeard's cap—French folktales were not for the faint-hearted (top right). Rumpelstiltskin—the Brothers Grimm knew how to spin a yarn (far right). ❧

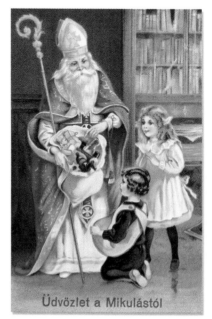

Üdvözlet a Mikulástól

In fact, one British newspaper has described them as the "first metrosexuals," favoring, as they did, well-groomed facial hair and beards that were plaited, waxed, and painstakingly trimmed. They also curled their mustaches and even dyed their beards to impress the fairer sex. This spilled over into the mythology they created, the Norse Sagas, in which the men all have beards and the women long hair. The beard in these tales was a potent symbol of virility, power, and wisdom. The hammer-wielding Norse god, Thor, is always described as red-bearded. When he is angry, he blows in his beard, setting off peals of thunder among the clouds.

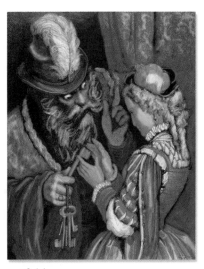

Beards are, of course, common in fairytales and folklore. Rumpelstiltskin has a long white beard in many versions of his tale, which originated in Germany and was collected by the Brothers Grimm. In their fairytale "King Grisly-beard," a beautiful but haughty princess is given the choice of a range of suitors but finds fault with every one, especially one with a beard "like an old mop," as she describes it. She is finally given in marriage to a scruffy fiddle player, who shows her the vast properties of Grisly-beard before taking her home to a life of drudgery. To the reader's amazement, it transpires that the fiddler and King Grisly-beard are one and the same! He has succeeded in curing her of pride, and the two marry and live happily and, in his case, hirsutely ever after.

But the tale of Bluebeard is probably the most famous tale involving a beard. The protagonist is a bearded aristocrat whose wives seem to disappear mysteriously. Horribly, their corpses are hidden away in a secret room, which is opened by his latest bride. Bluebeard meets his end when the brothers of his wife arrive. She inherits his castle and his fortune and forgets him. He lives on through his name, being used to describe a wife-murderer.

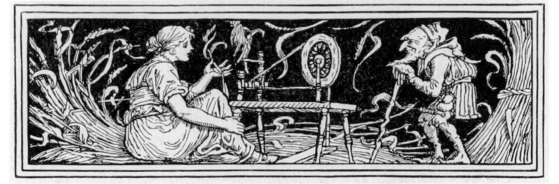

Art & Popular Culture

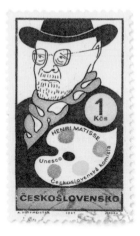

Masters of their Art
Czech postage stamp 1969 (top). Opposite, top row left to right: Charles Dickens, a barbershop quartet, Vincent van Gogh. Middle row left to right: Opera poster, Sir John Hurt photographed for Beard Season, *John Lennon. Bottom row left to right: Barber Shaun Dixon, Che Guevara, Dick Dastardly.* ❦

ONE HUNDRED YEARS before Instagram, troubled painter Vincent van Gogh mastered the art of the selfie. Almost always depicting himself with a distinctive russet beard, self-portraits of his chin clean-shaven are so rare that his "Self-Portrait without Beard" became one of the world's most expensive paintings when it was auctioned in the 1990s.

Facial hair has long been associated with disrupting social convention. Revolutionary, physician, motorcyclist, and beret-wearer Che Guevara is the quintessential icon of left-wing youthful rebellion. His reputation polarizes opinion, but his face, in the portrait *Guerrillero Heroico* by Alberto Korda, has been reproduced more than any other photographic image to date.

Aware of such connotations, British prime minister Margaret Thatcher once said she "wouldn't tolerate any minister of mine wearing a beard," yet in Victorian times Parliament bristled with bewhiskered politicians. Charles Dickens wrote a piece called "Why Shave?" exemplifying an age when the beard movement linked manliness to facial hair. Dickens wrote to a friend that without his glorious mustaches "life would be a blank," and his literary stardom had admiring fans emulating his "door-knocker" beard.

In the nineteenth century, whiskers had fabulously descriptive names including "thigh ticklers," "Piccadilly weepers," and "soup strainers." Indeed, the perils of consuming one's luncheon while eminently bearded were hotly debated. Perhaps such anxieties informed ex-Beatle John Lennon, who, a century later in Vienna, sang of "eating chocolate cake in a bag." His assertion that the most revolutionary thing you could do was to "stay in bed and grow out your hair" is forever associated with the 1970s peace movement, and his hirsute transformations from baby-faced mop-top to long-haired hippy, via the psychedelic Edwardian styling of Sgt. Pepper, were a barometer of the swiftly changing cultural landscape of the 1960s.

Actors routinely use facial hair to signify character type. The Beard Liberation Front named John Hurt as one of their Beards of the Year in 2013, when he became the first bearded Dr. Who and took part in Brock Elbank's *Beard*, a London photographic exhibition to raise awareness of the skin cancer charity Beard Season, founded by social media icon Jimmy Niggles.

As worn by wizards and Jedis, beards symbolize selfless wisdom. Cartoon villains, however, are mustachioed narcissists like "double-dealing do-badders" Boris Badenov, Snidely Whiplash, and racing driver Dick Dastardly. Based on British bounder Terry-Thomas in *Those Magnificent Men in their Flying Machines*, Dastardly's Mean Machine even has a nozzle that spreads mustache wax over the road to thwart his opponents.

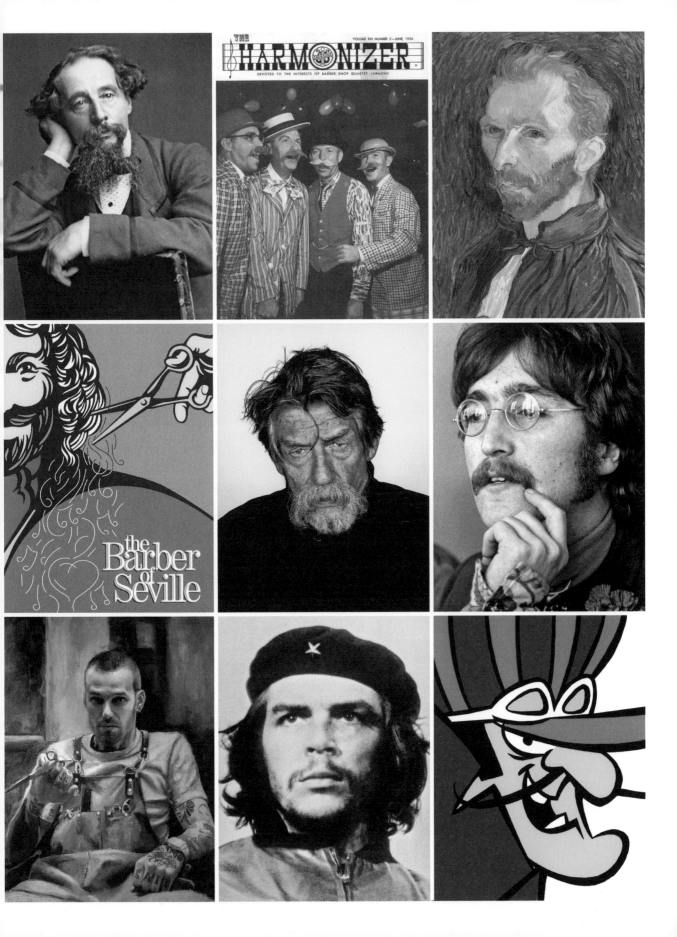

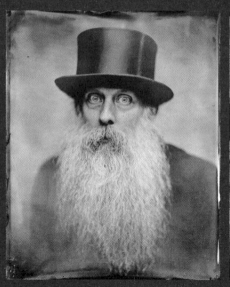

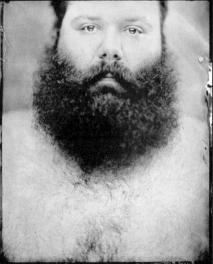

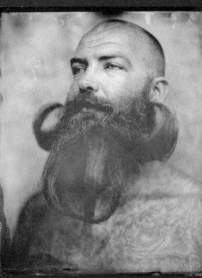

PROJECT BARBATYPE

Roger Fenton's 1880s images of hirsute soldiers fighting in the Crimea prompted a fashion for long beards. Project Barbatype uses the same historical process to create richly textured Tintypes, a handmade technology, to reflect the carnivalesque absurdity on display at modern beard competitions.

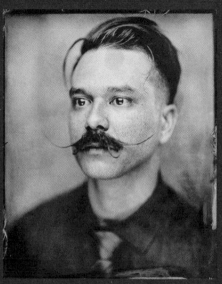

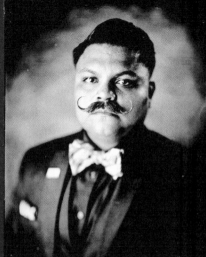

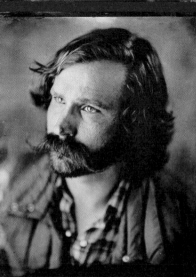

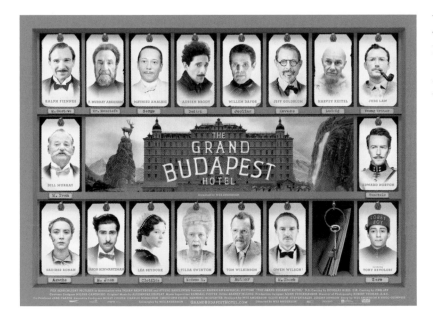

Waxing Lyrical
The Grand Budapest
Hotel *was styled with
Captain Fawcett products,
including the captain's very
own mustache wax (left).
One needs a mustache
"to be precise," says
Thompson (below).* ❧

Some cartoonists have a more affectionate view of mustaches. Tintin creator, Hergé, modeled clueless detective duo Thompson and Thomson on his father and uncle, identical twins who both had mustaches, dressed alike, and went out with walking canes or umbrellas, wearing bowler hats.

Sometimes barbers take center stage and not only when up to no good, like murderous Sweeney Todd. In 1813, Rossini, a wearer of splendid mutton chops, created *The Barber of Seville,* one of the great comic operas. With explosive vitality it tells the story of Figaro, a clever valet who stage-manages the action and became so popular its most famous aria was performed by Robin Williams, voicing a cartoon bird in the film *Mrs. Doubtfire.*

Grooming is an essential aspect of Wes Anderson's film *The Grand Budapest Hotel*, a stylized take on pre-World War II Europe with fabulous facial hair created by hair and make-up designer Frances Hannon. From Ralph Fiennes's neat waiter's mustache to Jeff Goldblum's beautifully conditioned Sigmund Freud number, the film is an undeniable hirsute treat.

In this age of the "rock star barber," London-based painter Vincent Kamp captures a series of tonsorial artists showcased in his 2017 exhibition *Cuts, Portraits of Barbers*. Today, it's not only hairstyles that command attention but also the people who create them and record them for posterity.

"Having his Ears Lowered"

After a brief Hollywood film career, the troubled and tragically short-lived James Dean went on to become a teenage icon. Posters showing his famous pompadour quiff graced the walls of many a fan following his death. A rebel without a cause still requires the services of a good barber.

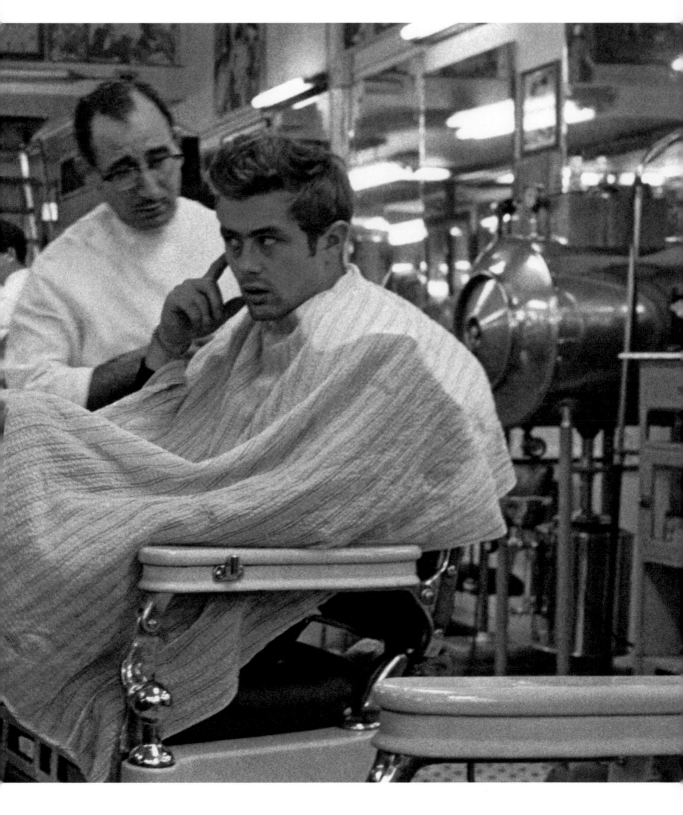

IVANA PRIMORAC

HAIR & MAKE-UP DESIGNER

*Born into an academic family in Croatia, Ivana Primorac eschewed the cap and gown to do something in which she was really interested. Her resumé now lists some of the best-loved movies of the last 25 years—*Spice World, Elizabeth, Gladiator, Billy Elliot, Cold Mountain, Sweeney Todd, The Reader, The Imitation Game, Steve Jobs ... *the list rolls on.*

I spoke to Ivana while she was engaged to design the hair and make-up for *The Crown*, the television blockbuster about the reign of Queen Elizabeth II. "It's got a lot of the same actors going through the 1930s to the 1960s. It will show the whole history of Her Majesty's reign and her 12 prime ministers. At the moment we are ending with Harold Macmillan. So there are a lot of different looks and people whose faces are familiar to us."

She tells of one fascinating snippet gleaned from the series: the little-known fact of a beard-growing competition instigated by Prince Philip while on a tour without the queen on the Royal Yacht *Britannia*. Every man on board grew his beard for three or four months. "It ended when a scandal broke out at home and Elizabeth called him to come back very quickly. In the meantime there's this footage of Philip on tour with a beard." The depiction of beard growth in stages, complementing the shooting schedule and, above all, looking realistic are typical of the challenges for the make-up department.

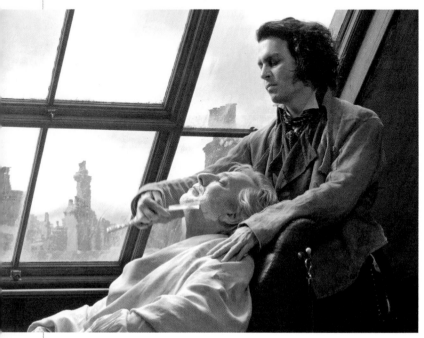

Sweeney Todd
Johnny Depp as the Demon Barber of Fleet Street wielding his cut-throat razor. Anyone for a slice of pie? ❦

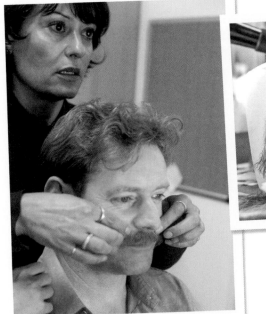
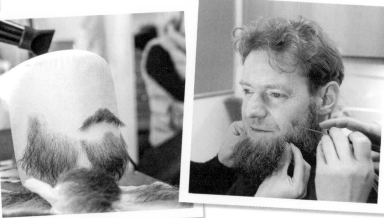

The Crowning Glory
Ivana painstakingly applying facial hair to aid the actor in his characterization. Are they ready for my close-up? ❧

Of course, hair and make-up also help the actors to find their character and express it appropriately. "Make-up and hair are a huge part of building a character for the actors. Quite often, if someone needs to look tired or distressed or upset or anything like that, facial hair serves that purpose very well because we know that people don't shave if they are in certain situations."

Lots of conventions can help you tell the story with facial hair. As for the process of creating the facial hair that can transport an actor to a different era or emotional state, it begins with consideration of the look. "You have to decide what look you want, how long you want it to

"FACIAL HAIR CAN TELL THE STORY OF A CHARACTER'S EMOTIONAL OR MENTAL STATE, OR IT MAY SIMPLY SERVE TO MAKE THEM LOOK MORE GROOMED OR MORE REGAL. YOU CAN MAKE SOMEONE LOOK MESSY AND UNTIDY, LIKE SOMEONE WHO HASN'T REALLY PAID ANY ATTENTION TO HIS APPEARANCE."

look, how groomed. Should it be natural? Should it be trimmed? You make those decisions and then you get the shape of someone's face. You do this by wrapping a bit of plastic wrap and stickytape around the face and then you draw their natural beard line on it. You take hair samples so you can tell the makers what shades of beard you'd like. It could have a bit more gray in it to look older. You send all that off to have it made. There're lots of technical decisions to be made. It can be in one or two pieces, for example. Then when it arrives, you have to know how to position and apply it. There's lots to working with facial hair."

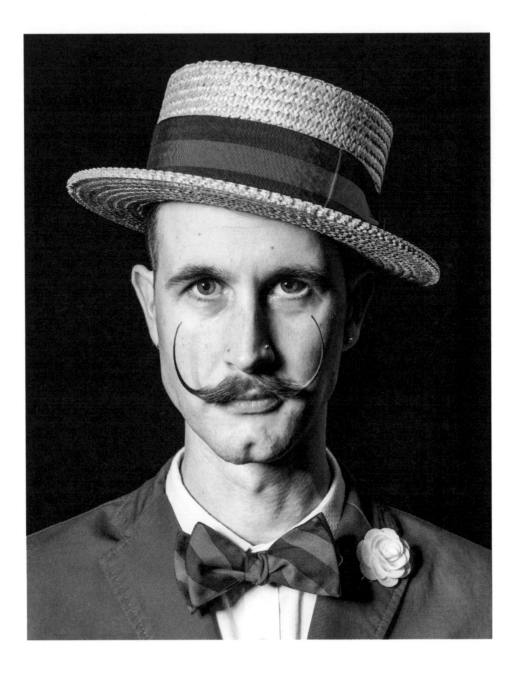

THE MODERN INDIVIDUAL

The modern gentleman's style is a witty celebration of global diversity. Well groomed and tailored, he puts a creative spin on respected traditions, making them his own. Such is the appearance of worldly wise men intent on blazing their own trail.

Selecting a Style

IT IS IMPOSSIBLE to pinpoint a fellow's individual style in the manner of a Victorian lepidopterist skewering specimen butterflies in a cabinet. Naturally, a chap might find his sartorial niche and sun himself there forever in blissful comfort, whereas others are more mercurial and flit from one look to another in the twirl of a waxed mustache. Some men live every minute adhering to a strict dress code, others adopt their attire as temporary costume for contests and gatherings, remodeling as the mood takes them. Whether a gentleman defies or defines a classification, society delights in neat distinctions, a mischievous moniker to describe the fashion of the time. Modern modes are eclectic, sourcing from one era to spruce up another, and it doesn't do to take oneself too seriously. While it is amusing to particularize, variations are certainly permissible. Indeed they are entirely desirable.

Gentlemen, like butterflies, are at their best when set free, and one should never underestimate the power of metamorphosis!

The Dapper Man

"Dapper"—a fine word with Germanic origins. Derived from the Dutch *dapper*, meaning brave, or the German word *tapfer*, meaning quick or courageous, it is defined in the Chambers Dictionary as "neat" or "spruce," which has an apt spring in its linguistic step. Since the first caveman painted his face with

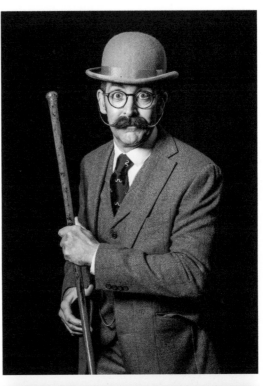

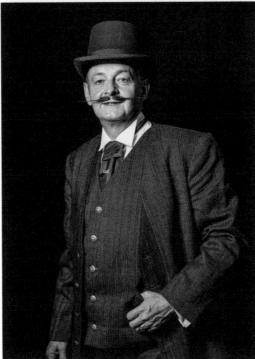

If You Want to Get Ahead, Get a Hat!
Johnny King (opposite), Allan Robinson (top), Bernd Hildebrandt (bottom). Headgear at a jaunty angle, a well-knotted necktie, boutonniere, and swagger stick are individual touches that complement this look. ❧

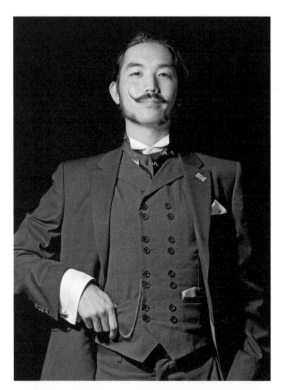

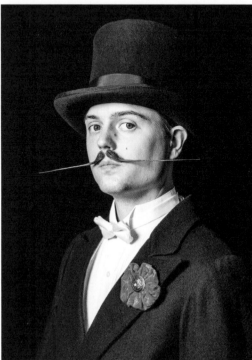

the latest in herbal dyes in order to attract a cavewoman, men have striven for the look that suits them. The Dapper Man is an expert in this field, a man who knows the difference between Harris and Donegal tweed (it's all in the provenance of the dyes and materials), who feels deeply the assurance of a metal collar stud, and who is au fait with the topiary of his nasal hair. He may even make use of a foot grater, just in case he has to don his $500 Tom Ford leather sandals. His watch will be the right one for the occasion, and it may even tell the time.

Of course, the Dapper Man will have an exquisite vintage shaving kit—maybe even a Gillette 24-carat-gold adjustable "Fatboy" safety razor—or if he has a hirsute visage, as well he might, he will indulge in exquisite unctions from the stable of Captain Fawcett or any other good purveyor of first-class gentleman's grooming requisites.

The Young Fogey
Coined by British journalist Alan Watkins, writing in *The Spectator* magazine in 1984, the humorous term Young Fogey refers to a rather buttoned-down individual, conservative in his tastes and something of an aesthete in his lifestyle.

His dress style is vintage, usually referring to the 1920s and '30s, the era of the "bright, young things" immortalized in Evelyn Waugh's *Vile Bodies*. The style is a little shabby chic, heavy tweeds of the sort gentlemen in the

Jolly Good Fellows
*Philip G. W. Smith (top), Patrick Fette (bottom).
Further image punctuation might include a finely waxed mustache, wing-tipped collar, and starched shirt fronts, an ascot, and a pair of cufflinks.* ❧

1920s sported when they went to a country house party. Think *Downton Abbey* but 95 years later. Dinner jackets would be decidedly antique, and the Young Fogey might even be seen in a smoking jacket as he takes his leisure at home, smoking his pipe and sipping a cheeky little Montrachet. Hair is short and oiled with a parting as clearly defined as his politics—probably on the right side—and the Young Fogey's chin is shaved to within an inch of its life.

The early devotees, to whom Watkins was refering, were writers, artists, journalists, and poets with a taste for the halcyon days of the interwar years. A number of students at some of the older universities might aspire to this style, and adherents can be found sprinkled across professions such as law, antiquarian book dealing, and tailoring.

The Mountain Man

What does it take to create the look of the mountain man? Think Grizzly Adams in the late 1970s television series *The Life and Times of Grizzly Adams*. Huge beard because you live in a shack in the wild, not a first-floor, centrally heated apartment in Greenwich Village; thick, down jacket—perhaps buckskin—and heavy boots. Lots of plaid or tartan flannel work shirts—the Mountain Man can never have too many flannel shirts. Chunky button sweaters or cardigans are needed for those chilly nights on the mountain or for dining alfresco in SoHo. Thick denims are de rigueur, and hair

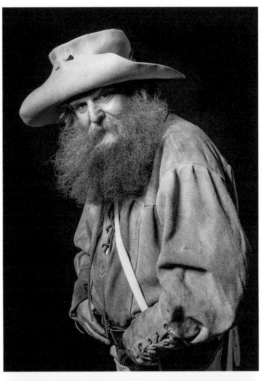

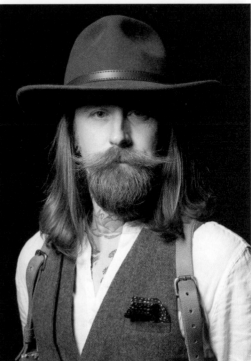

No Axe to Grind

"Fuzzy" (top), Aaron Jamie (bottom). Alternatively one may adopt a more rugged look, albeit apparently less contrived. Adherents dress in work-wear clothes made from materials such as leather, canvas, plaid, and denim. ❧

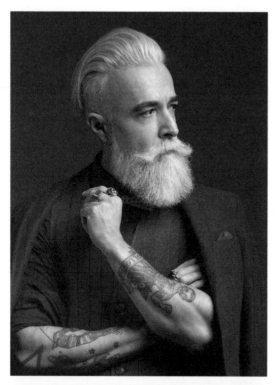

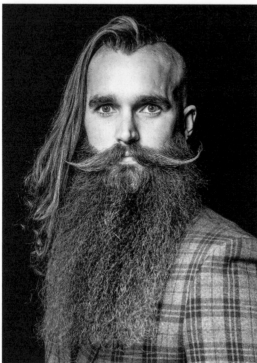

should be long and straggly, as if it has been a stranger to the comb for a few weeks.

The Hipster

The Hipster first donned his thrift-store-purchased, checked shirt and expensively distressed boots in newly gentrified areas of the world's style capitals—first, probably, in Williamsburg in New York City and then in London's Shoreditch, the 3rd Arrondissement of Paris, Berlin's Kreuzberg and Prenzlauer Berg, and Stockholm's Södermalm, at the turn of the 21st century.

The term originates in the 1940s, being used to describe young people who were trendily dressed, but today it encompasses a whole lot more than well-maintained beards, sculpted staches, tight jeans, Mr. Magoo glasses, and drinking cocktails out of Mason jars. He may wear his hair slicked back as the counterpoint to a bushy beard, or there can be a messy top and shorn sides. Pompadours have time-traveled from the 1950s, and the man-bun can often be seen on a skateboard or bicycle.

Where might one find such a chap? Working in the world of media or design, perhaps. Or as an entrepreneur, opening a micro-brewery, a café selling 120 different breakfast cereals from around the world, or, perhaps, a company making the very mustache wax and beard balm they lavish on themselves.

All Hail the Hirsute!
Alessandro Manfredini (top), Maxwell Newton (bottom). Brock Elbank's iconic image of Jimmy Niggles, the founder of Beard Season (opposite). ❧

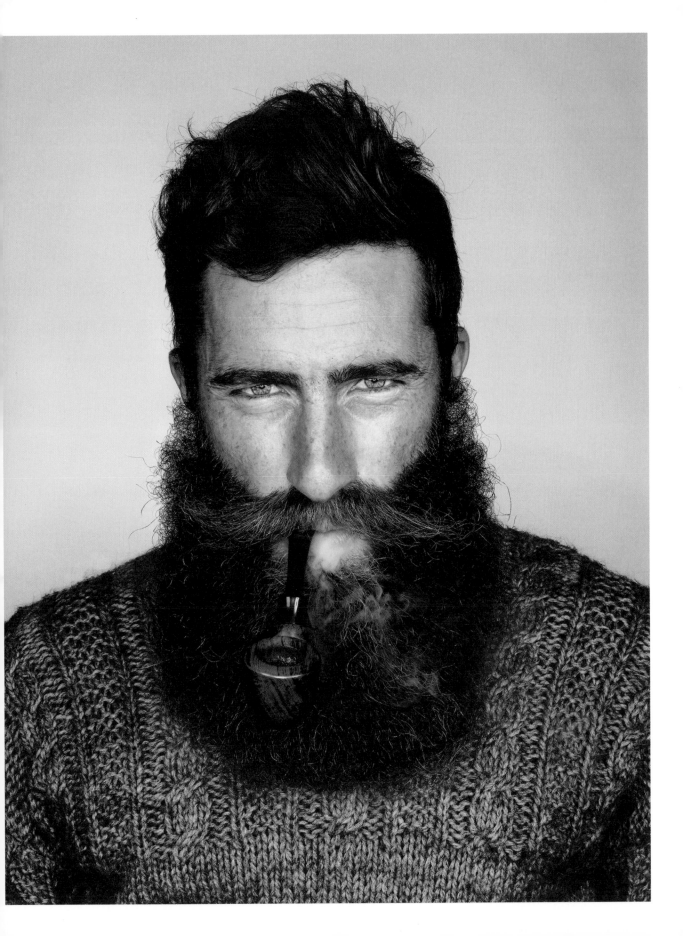

The Biker

The biker first roared into the public consciousness on his 1950 Triumph Thunderbird 6T with the release of the 1953 film *The Wild One*. Marlon Brando, playing the leader of the Black Rebels Motorcycle Club, was asked by a local worthy, "What are you rebelling against?" and famously replied, "Whaddaya got?"

Motorcycle clubs had been around in some form since the 1920s, and the most well known of them all, the Hells Angels, was founded on March 17, 1948. Men returning from World War II, craving the camaraderie they had enjoyed in the forces, formed motorcycle groups and often bestowed names on these clubs that reflected the squadrons or fighting groups they had been part of during the conflict. Indeed, one of the squadrons of the Flying Tigers (1st American Volunteer Group) of the Chinese Air Force in 1941–42 went by the name of "Hell's Angels."

Brando's sneering existentialism launched an entire style borrowed from real bikers: a leather-jacketed, tight-jeaned look with greasy hair slicked back with pomade. The look took off and was—and still is—emulated around the world. Later, the look was purloined in part by the Village People. The hyper-masculine Leatherman Biker was one of the most popular and helped to popularize a look among S&M gay men that involved leather, prodigious sideburns, and a long, bushy Zapata-style mustache.

Traditionally seen as part of an anti-establishment counter-culture, bikers often wear spectacular beards and long hair as well as plentiful tattoos and piercings.

Full Throttle!
Two hirsute chaps at Wheels and Waves, Biarritz (below).
Marlon Brando as Johnny Strabler (opposite). ✺

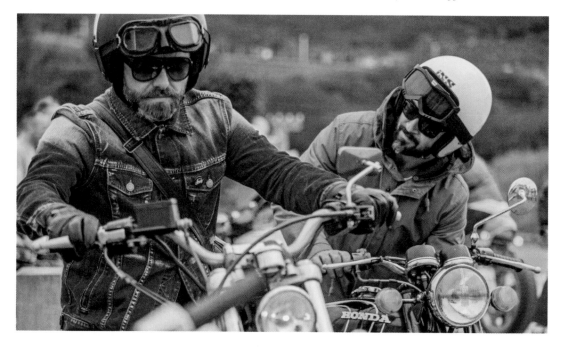

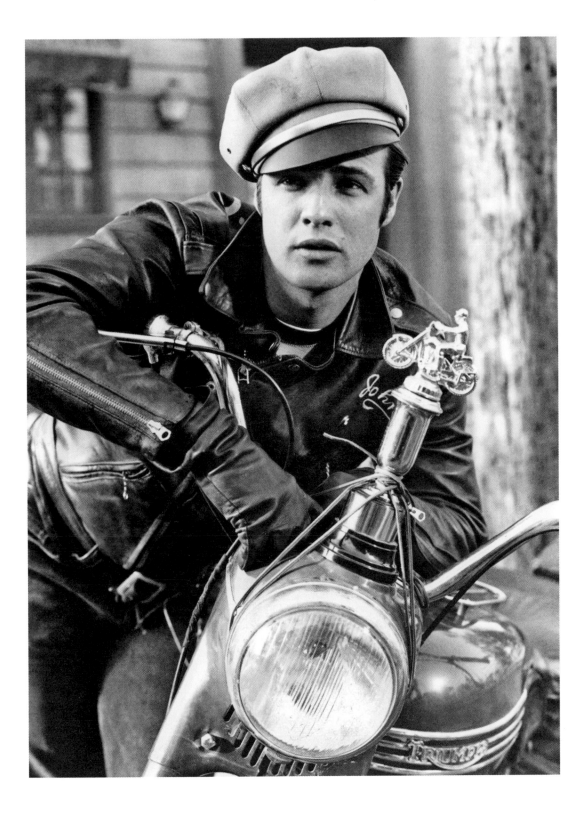

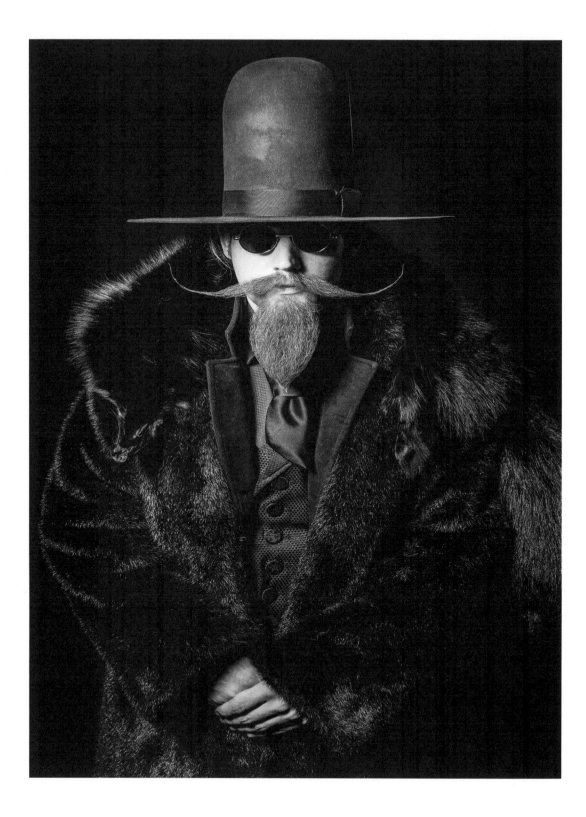

Steampunk

In the late 1980s, writer K. W. Jeter allegedly came up with "Steampunk" to describe his own work, and the term has expanded from a subdivision of science fiction and fantasy to cover an entire lifestyle, ranging from music and fashion to literature and engineering.

The fashions of the nineteenth and early twentieth centuries are riotously plundered to create a style reinventing modern technologies and splicing them with an alternative Industrial Revolution. Revelling in elaborate detailing, from lace and leather to spikes and frills, it is the romantic cousin of dystopian cyberpunk expressed with a gritty operatic mechanical elegance.

Authors Jules Verne and H. G. Wells are undoubted heroes, but the backdrop of Victorian England is redrawn with a non-conformist punk aesthetic. *Chitty Chitty Bang Bang* meets *Mad Max*, *Blade Runner* meets *Bagpuss*. Pieces one might uncover in a junk shop—cogs and crystals, brass goggles and taxidermy specimens—are handsomely reimagined and incorporated into styling that explores the integration of man and machine, science and the occult. There is a touch of fetish, a whisper of goth, a shake of burlesque, and a dash of the military. Lace and velvet, top hats and tweed, pith helmets and capes all combine, and there is always a whiff of an eccentric inventor's oil in the air. Steampunk is a creative declaration of individualism for the modern time-traveling gentleman.

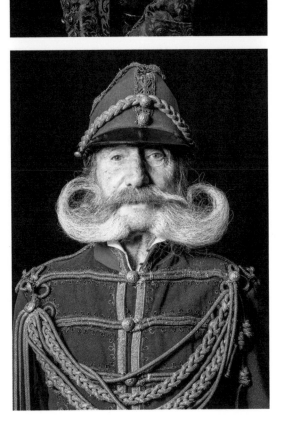

Anachronistic Dandies
Jeffrey Moustache (opposite), James Barker (top), Bruno Panza (bottom). The rules are there are no rules. ❧

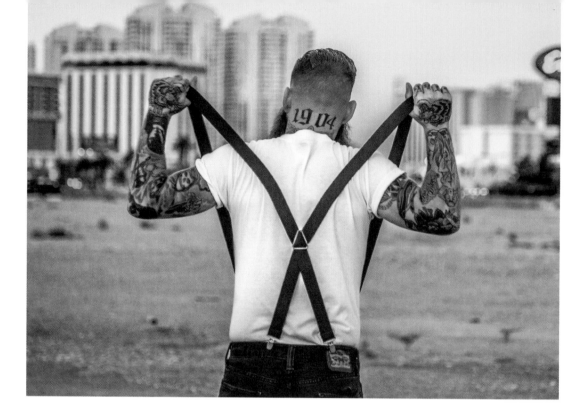

The Tattooed Man

The word "tattoo" derives from the Polynesian word *tatau*, meaning "to write," but prior to its coining, tattooing had been known to the West as painting, scarring, or staining. The first description of tattoos can be found in the journal of Joseph Banks, the naturalist on Captain Cook's vessel, HMS *Endeavour*. He wrote: "I shall now mention the way they mark themselves indelibly, each of them is so marked by their humour or disposition." Cook himself refers to the "tattaw."

Many cultures have practiced tattooing. Tattoos decorated the faces of the Ainu, an indigenous Japanese tribe, as well as those of peoples of Taiwan, the Berbers of North Africa, the Hausa, Yoruba, and Fulani of Nigeria, and, most notably, the Maori of New Zealand. The Maori call their distinctive face and body marking Tā moko, and it traditionally differs from the tattoo in that the skin is carved by chisels known as uhi, rather than punctured by a needle or sharp implement.

Tattooing has been practiced throughout history all over the world, including in the United Kingdom. In fact, it has been suggested that the name of Great Britain owes something to the art. "Britons" translates as "people of the designs" or "painted people" and refers to the Picts of the north of the island.

There are countless reasons for getting a tattoo. It could be an acknowledgment of love for another person; it could mark a rite of passage, a religious symbol, a talisman, status or rank; it may represent an act of bravery by the wearer or a simple aesthetic statement. There have been less desirable tattoos, of course—as punishment, for example, or to signify the wearer's status as a convict or slave.

The tattoo was long viewed as undesirable, worn by ex-cons, sailors, and people on the margins of society. Now, having some ink on your body is almost de rigueur. Even the actress Dame Judi Dench has one. At the age of 81 she had "carpe diem" tattooed on her wrist.

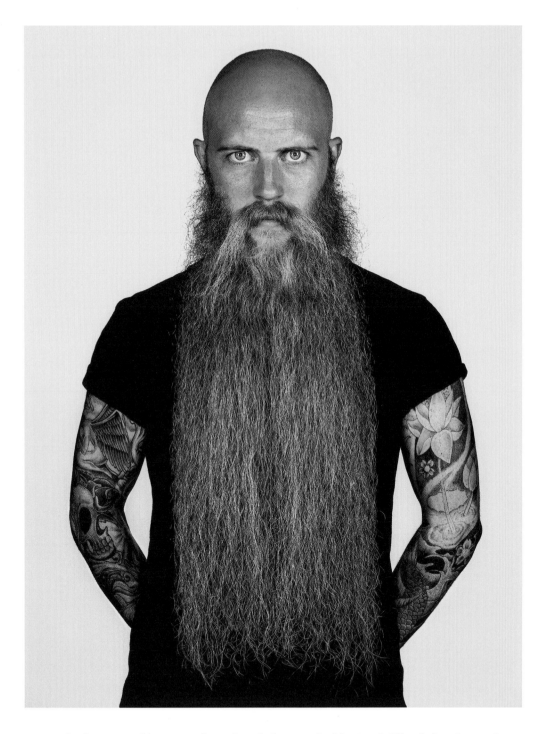

Michael Legge and his magnificent beard photographed by Brock Elbank for #Project60 in support of the skin cancer charity Beard Season. Very well done, gentlemen!

RICKI HALL
GENTLEMAN & DANDY

After a chance meeting at the Ritzy Cinema in Brixton, I developed a firm friendship with Ricki and work with him in producing his range of grooming products.

Ricki Hall is one of the world's top models, having starred in numerous campaigns for brands such as Diesel, H&M, David Beckham, TJ Maxx, and Paul Smith, among others, and he has graced the covers and pages of magazines worldwide. Instantly recognizable from his abundant dark beard and a collection of distinctive tattoos, he has an unlikely background for a model. After leaving school at 15, he went to work in the family motorbike shop. In his early 20s, on a daytrip to London, he was spotted by a model scout. "At the time I had a slicked-back mohawk, and one arm was tattooed, and I had this big Freddie Mercury mustache. She told me she was really interested in my look and asked me if I fancied being a model. I thought she was having a joke, but she put me in a taxi, took me to the agency, and they signed me straight away. I had to move down to London almost immediately because Fashion Week was coming up and they were doing the casting. So, that's how I became a model."

> "MY STYLE HAS EVOLVED FROM A FLASHY LITTLE HOOLIGAN WHEN I WORKED AT MY DAD'S BIKE SHOP, TO 1950S NEW YORK WORK WEAR, TO '70S-INSPIRED FLORAL OPEN SHIRTS WITH HIPPY LONG HAIR."

That Ricki looked different from other models at the time gave him the edge. "I've always been interested in art, and with that comes an interest in tattoos. I've been an avid tattoo collector since I was seventeen. The beard came from when I first moved down to London and had absolutely no money whatsoever. All I had were the clothes on my back, a bag of bits and bobs, and that was it. I was sofa-surfing and working in a shop in Camden, the Happy Shack. It was a really badly paid job, and I couldn't afford a razor or shaving gear. So, I just let my beard grow, and that's how that came about, out of pure laziness and because I was broke! When I had been growing it for a while I popped into my agency to pick up some pictures for my model book, and they took a look at me and liked what they saw. They decided to put me forward for casting for a campaign by Lyle & Scott, the Scottish menswear company, and I got the job. It was my first campaign, and that was what put me on the map."

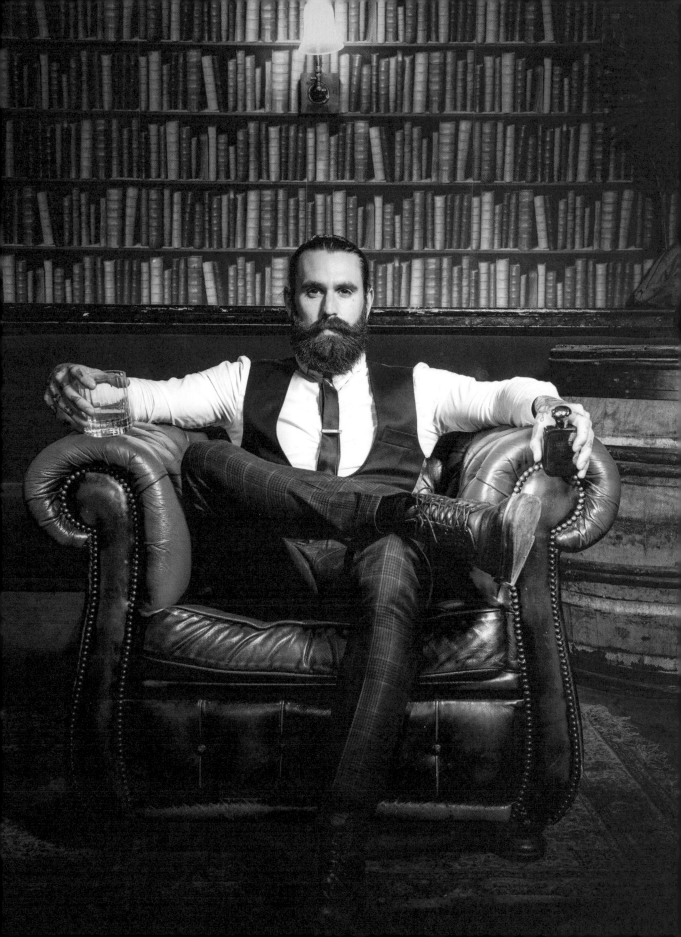

THE BIG SHAVE

In 2016, Ricki made the monumental decision to have his beard shaved off. He did it to raise awareness for Mesothelioma U.K., following his father's death from the disease.

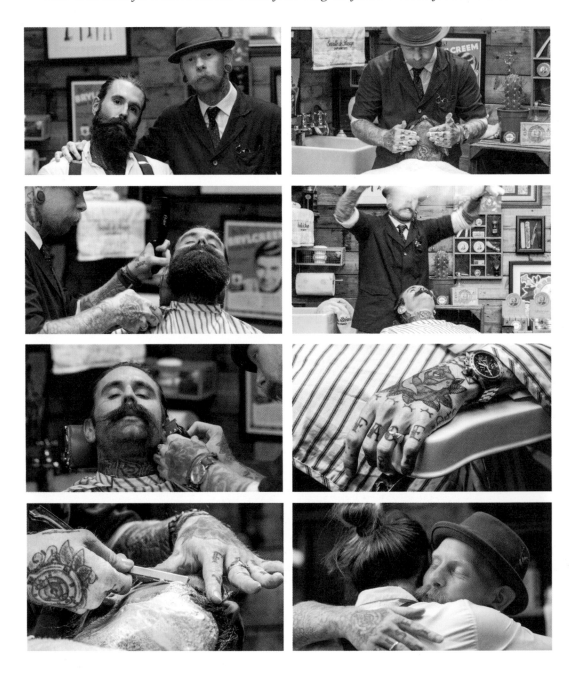

Clean Faced

Mesothelioma is a cancer associated with exposure to asbestos, and Ricki's father contracted it when working in factories when he was about 20. Ricki explains: "It's getting quite common now because it takes about 40 years for this cancer to show its ugly face. I'm doing everything I can to raise awareness and money. When I had the beard shaved off by Frank Rimer at Thy Barber in Shoreditch, we raised around £7,000. I hadn't seen my face for so long and I looked so young, although I did still have a massive Daniel Day-Lewis Gangs of New York mustache.'

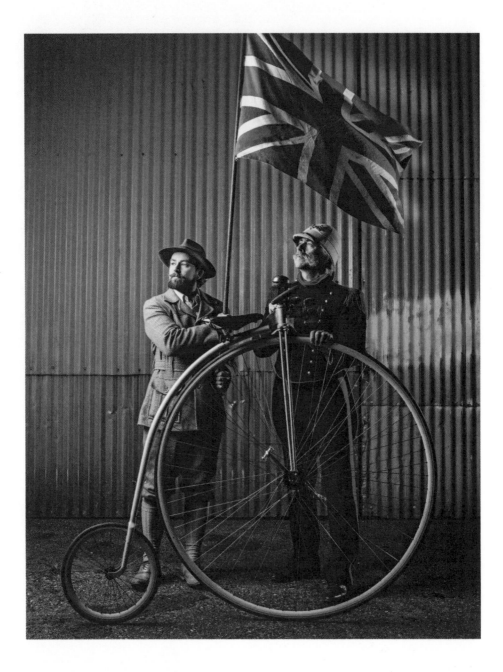

GENTLEMANLY GATHERINGS

*The modern gentleman's calendar is chockablock with a whole host of to see and
be seen at events, a chance to mingle with fellow natty dressers who are waxed
and pomaded to the hilt. Distinguished is as distinguished does!*

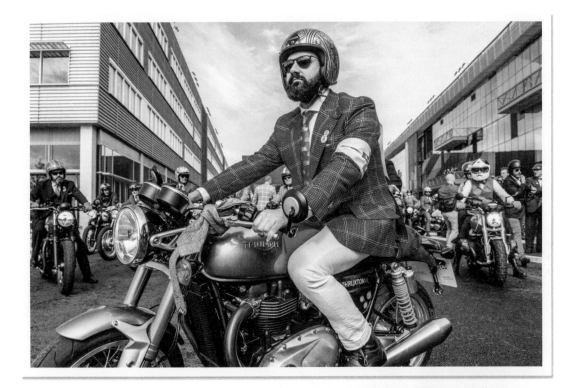

Celebrating the Beard

FROM PARAGUAY TO Pakistan, from Northern Ireland to South Korea, gentlemen congregate at a number of events to preen, promenade, and parade. One might roll up in a gleaming sports car, pedal by on a restored bicycle, or speed off astride a custom café racer. Others simply stroll up shod in handmade brogues, occasionally displaying their latest ink.

Often aligned with a specific charity or very worthy cause, such social gatherings are an opportunity to shake one's well groomed tail feathers and have a splendid time in like-minded convivial company.

Two Wheels Are Better Than One
Alistair Cope of Velo Vintage (opposite). Mark Hawwa, founder of the Distinguished Gentleman's Ride (above). ❦

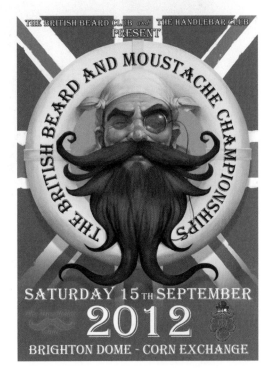

THE BRITISH BEARD CLUB *and* THE HANDLEBAR CLUB
PRESENT

THE BRITISH BEARD AND MOUSTACHE CHAMPIONSHIPS

SATURDAY 15TH SEPTEMBER
2012
BRIGHTON DOME · CORN EXCHANGE

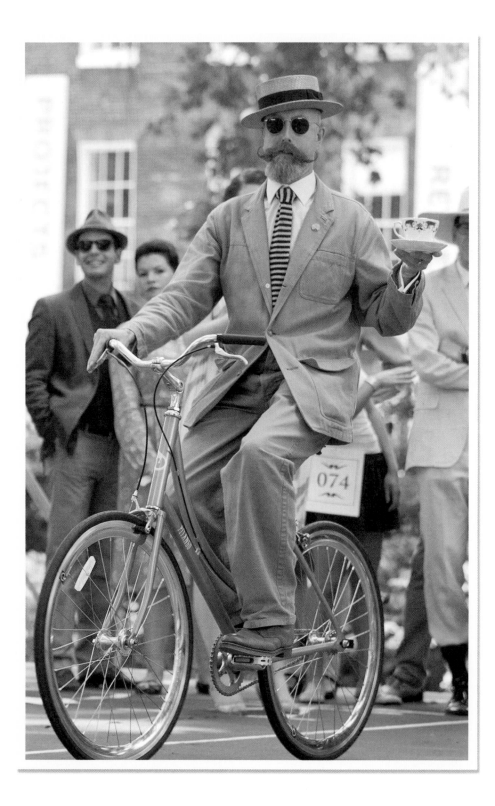

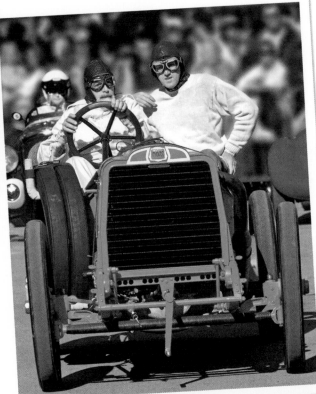

THE GOODWOOD REVIVAL

A historic race meeting staged at Lord March's country estate, the Goodwood Revival celebrates both the romance and period glamour of motor racing during its heyday (left). ❧

THE DISTINGUISHED GENTLEMAN'S RIDE

Mark Hawwa founded the DGR after seeing a picture of Mad Men's *Don Draper dressed in his nattiest suit, astride a classic motorbike. Now every year tens of thousands of people wax their mustaches and oil their beards before donning their helmets and heading out on their classic and vintage motorcycles to raise funds for health charities (below).* ❧

THE CHAP OLYMPIAD

Hosted by British magazine The Chap *every year in a central London square, the Chap Olympiad is less a sporting event than a celebration of the modern gentleman (opposite). As the organizers say, "More points are awarded for maintaining immaculate trouser creases than crossing the finishing line."* ❧

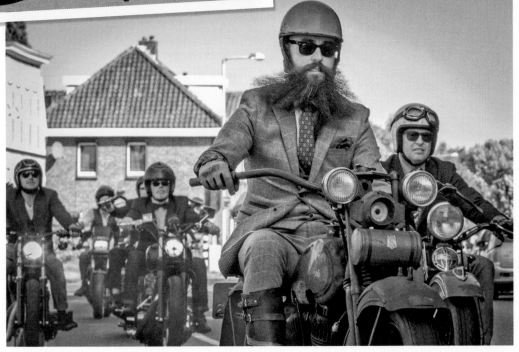

DIARY DATES FOR THE MAN ABOUT TOWN

A sample of suggested social events

APRIL

WESSEX BEARDSMEN

The Wessex Beard & Mustache competition is one of the first must-be-seen-at social events of the year. It is typical of an ever-increasing number of charitable beard and mustache related gatherings hosted by regional "thatches," often under the auspices of the British Beard Club. *All hail the hirsute!*

MAY

THE TWEED RUN

A annual bicycle ride through the streets of London. Attracting hundreds of snappily dressed cyclists who bowl along in their vintage best with the occasional stop for tea and cake. *Press on!*

JUNE
ROYAL ASCOT

A long-established highlight in the British horse-racing calendar, an event that requires a strict dress code and is synonymous with sartorial elegance. Famed for "Hooray Henrys," extravagant millinery, and lashings of Champagne. *Tally ho!*

JULY

HENLEY REGATTA

A major rowing event first held in 1839 on the River Thames. For those not messing about in boats, it's an ideal opportunity to see and be seen while quaffing Pimms, attired in your very best blazer and flannels. *What ho!*

CHAP OLYMPIAD

A tongue-in-cheek celebration having a laugh at athletic endeavor. Taking place in a leafy London square, it gives one the chance to demonstrate accomplishments such as mixing martinis without the aid of a butler, and the ability to toss a cucumber sandwich with an air of panache.

Attracting "anarcho-dandies," this is an occasion where one might be chastised for not having properly creased trousers. *Toodle pip!*

AUGUST

ASYLUM STEAMPUNK FESTIVAL

Held in Lincoln Castle and its immediate environs, it's a riotous assembly, an eclectic mix of the dispossessed that includes Victorian science fantasists, time travelers, and a smattering of fringe lunatics. Dress as you see fit, the weirder and wackier the better. *Time for tea dueling!*

SEPTEMBER

WORLD BEARD & MUSTACHE CHAMPIONSHIPS

This biennial competition has been held previously in locations as diverse as Carson City, Brighton, Anchorage, Trondheim, Leogang, and Austin. With strict judging in up to 18 different categories, the prizes are fiercely contested by some of the world's greatest exponents of facial hair. *Shave it for later!*

GOODWOOD REVIVAL

A veritable *Boys' Own* event that appeals to the engine geek in us all. It's a concentration of some of the world's greatest motorcycles, vintage autos, and flying machines punctuated by the evocative aroma of hot Castrol. It's a chance for you to wear period dress and pit your wits while racing on this classic circuit. *Chocks away, chaps!*

LONDON TATTOO CONVENTION

One of the best alternative gatherings on the circuit, showcasing some of the very best skin artists at work. As gentlemen have done since time immemorial, wear your ink with pride. *Tattoo you, sir!*

OCTOBER

BRITISH BEARD & MUSTACHE CHAMPIONSHIPS

Held biennally, previous contests have taken place in Brighton, Bath, and Liverpool, with the next event scheduled to take place in 2018.

Competition categories include:
Mustache *English, Dalí, Handlebar, Mustache Freestyle*
Partial Beard *Natural Goatee, Musketeer, Chops, Partial Beard Freestyle*
Full Beard *Verdi, Garibaldi, Natural Full Beard, Full Beard Freestyle*
This is a simply splendid opportunity to raise money for charity while displaying extravagantly styled facial hair. *Britain at its best!*

THE HANDLEBAR CLUB

Founded in 1947 in a dressing room of the Windmill Theatre, London, this is a mustache-only club, with beards strictly prohibited. Monthly meetings are held somewhere in west London, usually in a convivial pub, with the only sport allowed being the playing of darts. Word has it that ladies are now being admitted, which is, after all, entirely in keeping with the club's inaugural meeting when the founders were minuted as being outnumbered by showgirls. *Ooh matron!*

NOBLE CAUSES

Beard Season

Originally founded in Australia by Jimmy Niggles as a tribute to his friend Wes Bonny, lost to melanoma. Beard Season is now a global campaign promoting skin cancer awareness. You simply grow your beard as a conversation starter, have a skin check enabling early cancer detection, and encourage others to do the same. Grow on!

The Distinguished Gentleman's Ride

The DGR is a global motorcycle fundraising event that promotes awareness of prostate cancer and male suicide prevention. Participants ride classic, old school café racers and bobbers while adopting a dapper dress code and conducting themselves in an affable manner. In 2016 the Ride attracted more than 50,000 bikers in over 500 cities across 90 countries. Start your engines!

Movember

Movember started in 2003 and encourages men to grow a mustache in the month of November. The charity harnessed social media, creating a global community. To date it has raised over £400 million and funded more than 1,200 men's health projects. Well done, chaps!

Decembeard

A U.K. charity that encourages men to grow beards and set up light-hearted social fundraising events with the serious aim of beating bowel cancer. Being in December, these events often have a festive flavor. A veritable winter warmer!

ALICE JELLEY
CHAMPIONSHIP JUDGE

I first encountered Alice Jelley at a Steampunk festival. It was at that point that she realized she wanted to learn more about the competitive world of facial hair, and she's since gone on to judge the weird and wonderful at the British Championships.

Alice's first encounter with a facial hair club was while on vacation in Texas. She drove to the state's capital city, Austin, and joined the guys and girls of the Austin Facial Hair Club at one of their "Meat & Greets." Fortified with a Lone Star beer and some brisket, Alice found everyone to be warm and welcoming, and she instantly felt among friends. Since then she has attended many competitions in the U.K. and in Austria, and in various states. Alice helps her friend Victoria run BILF—Beard I'd Like to Fondle, an apparel company raising funds for worthy causes. In 2014, at the British Beard & Mustache Championships, she won the ladies' handmade fake category with her "Everything's Bigger in Texas" beard, a tribute to her friends in Austin.

Alice explains, "In 2016 the British Championships were hosted by the Liverbeards at St. George's Hall in Liverpool. Rather than enter the competition I was asked to help in the organization and running of the event, having gained a great deal of knowledge and experience from other competitions globally. I recruited the judges for the day, and BILF did the pre-judging. Generally the size of the competition denotes how many categories there are going to be. For example, the smaller 'thatch' competitions, such as the annual one hosted by the Wessex Beardsmen, will not have as many categories as the British or the World Championships. In this year's British Championships we had an under 1 inch freestyle category (measured from the chin) which was my favorite. Some people may be surprised at this, but I believe it allowed people who are new to growing their beard to get involved with our amazing facial hair world. We had guys who had just walked in off the street who entered this category." Alice points out that there might be guys who because of their jobs are not allowed to have a long beard and therefore need to keep it short. This category enabled them to participate.

"Last but by no means least are the fake categories. They are for anyone who would like to make a fake beard and/or mustache. It can be split into kids and adults or can be just for the ladies as a 'Whiskerina' category. But it can also be split into a natural style whereby you make the facial hair look as realistic as possible or a creative style whereby you can make facial hair out of anything and everything."

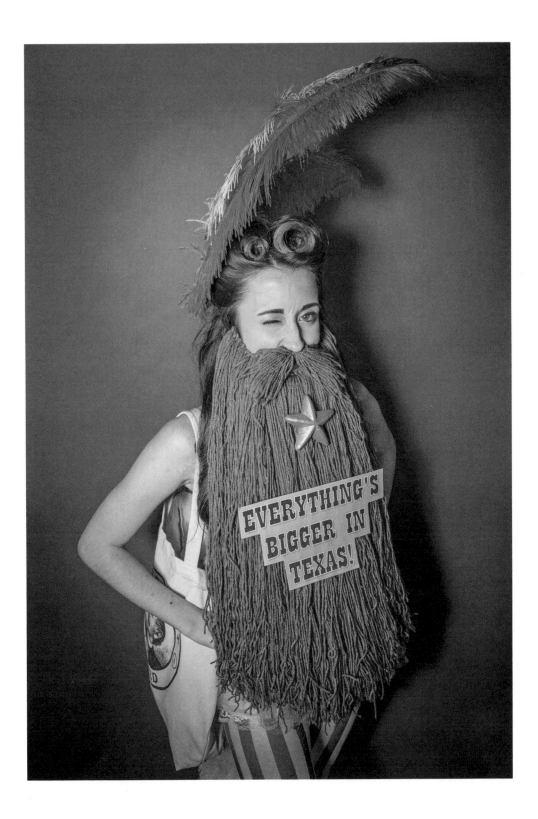

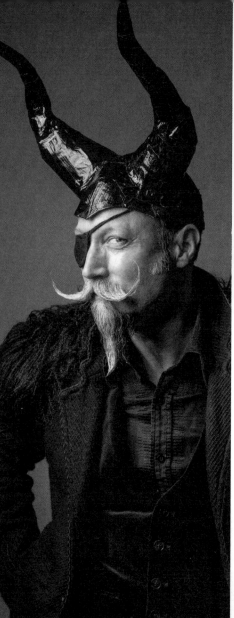

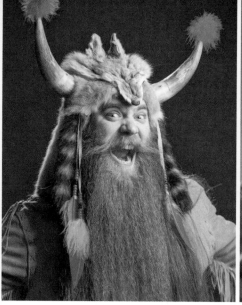

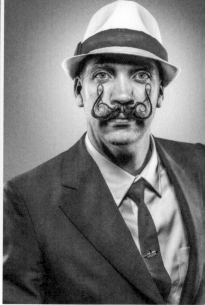

FABULOUS FACIAL DISPLAYS

In the course of my wanderings, it has been my great privilege to document a panoply of hirsute gentlemen displaying their own unique sartorial style. The vital impulse these men share is their passion for the creative cultivation of facial hair. Please allow me to present a veritable gallery of ruggedly resplendent rogues!

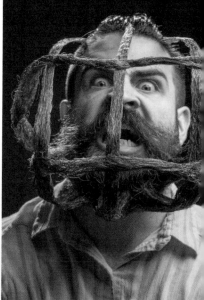

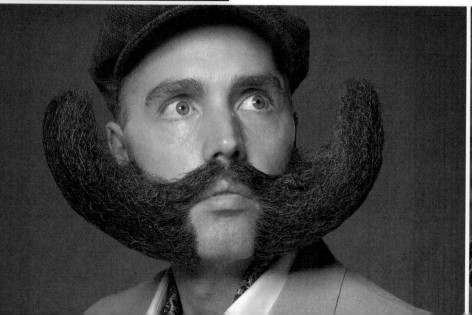

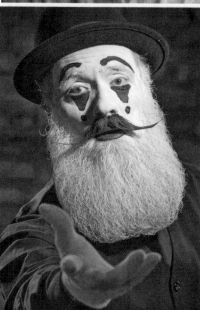

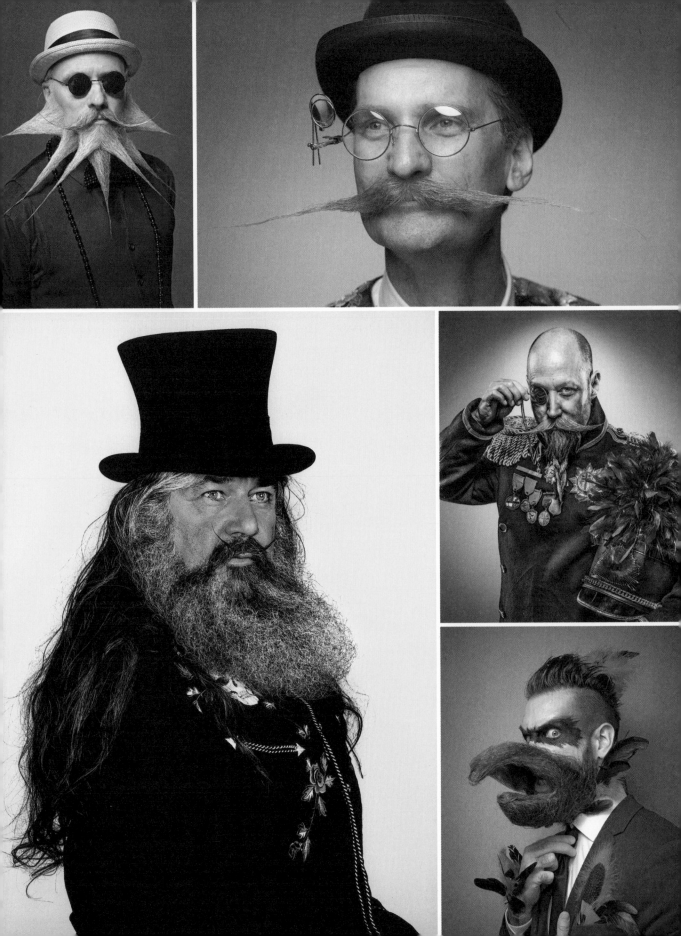

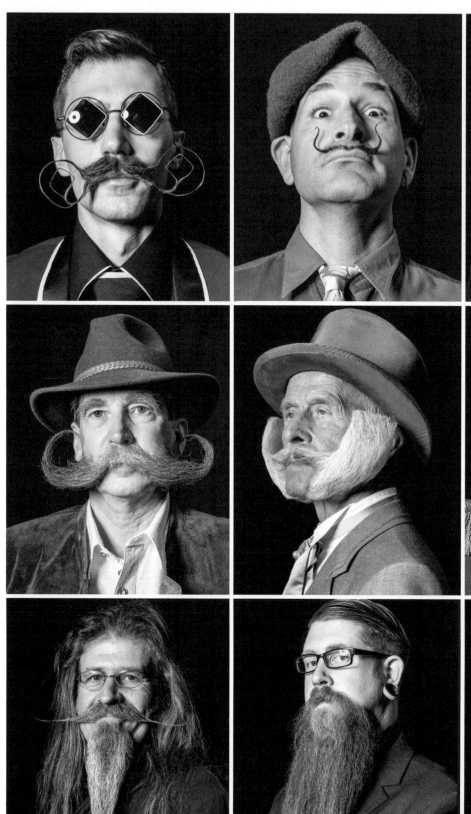
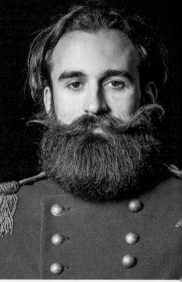
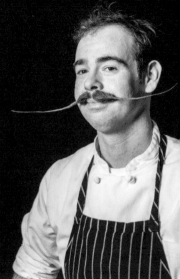

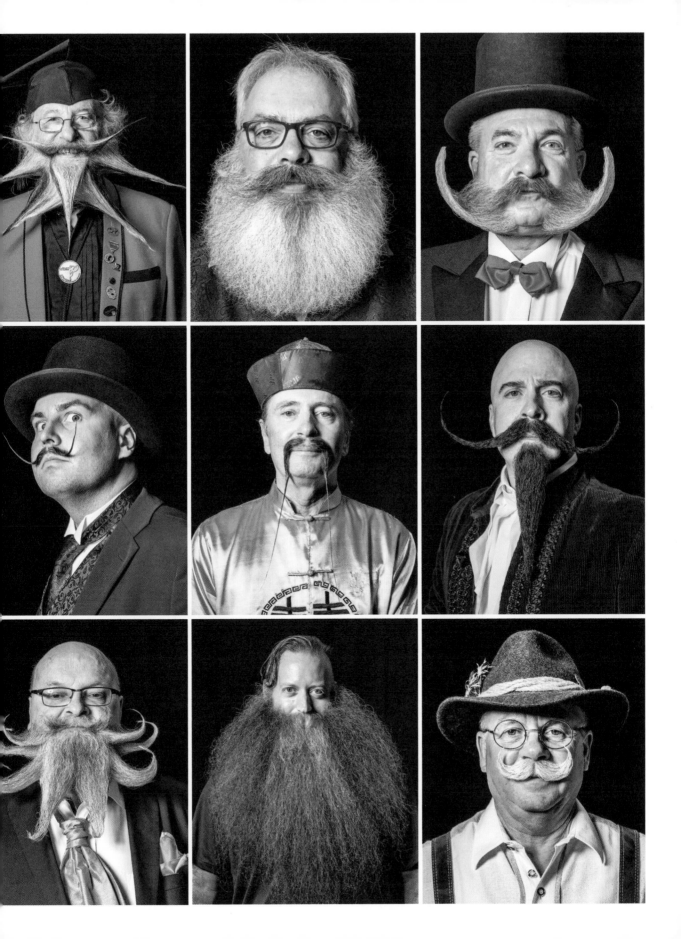

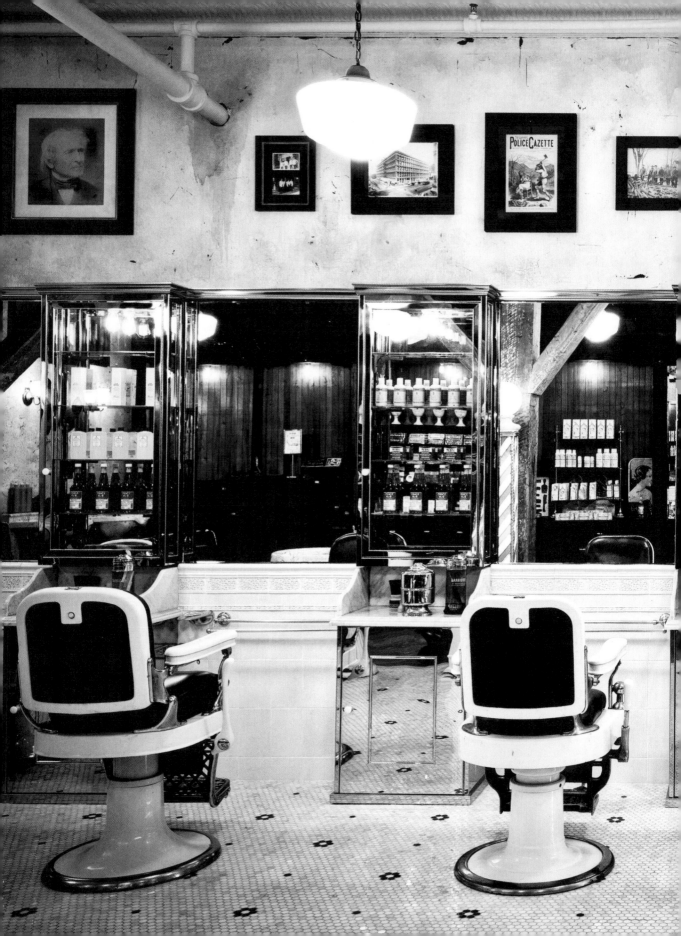

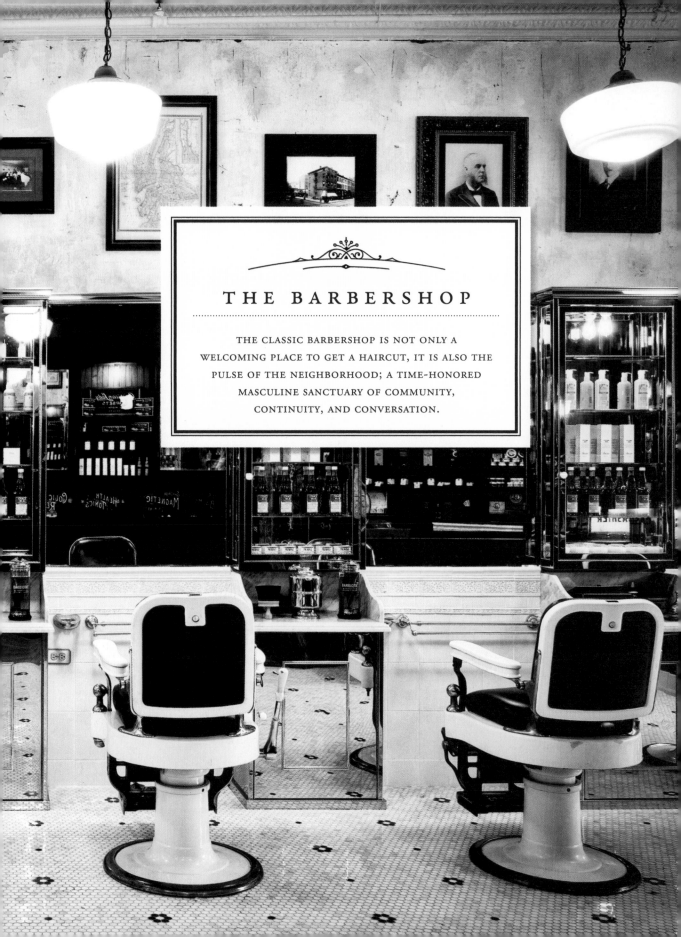

THE BARBERSHOP

THE CLASSIC BARBERSHOP IS NOT ONLY A
WELCOMING PLACE TO GET A HAIRCUT, IT IS ALSO THE
PULSE OF THE NEIGHBORHOOD; A TIME-HONORED
MASCULINE SANCTUARY OF COMMUNITY,
CONTINUITY, AND CONVERSATION.

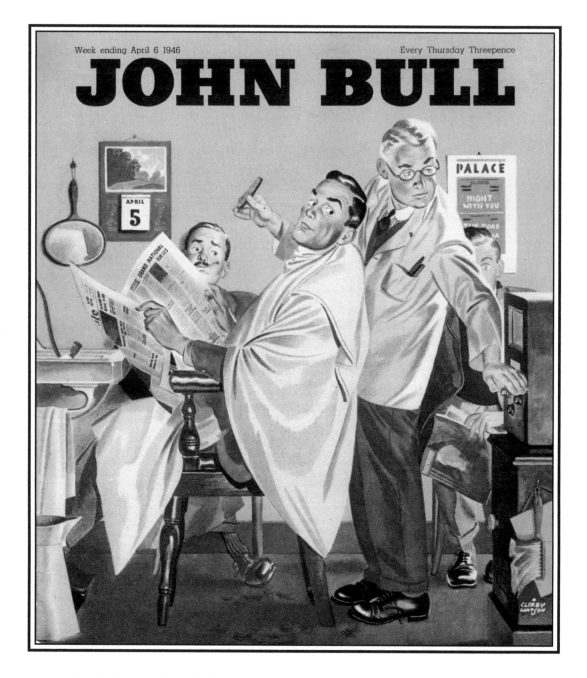

Founded in 1906 by Liberal MP Horatio Bottomley, John Bull *encapsulated post-war Britain and employed some of Britain's finest illustrators.*

ONE LIKES HAVING to keep up with new-fangled contraptions. Indeed, my own emporium utilizes the modern wonder of the worldwide Web, keeping an elegant finger on the global pulse. However, the most important things in life may not be purchased online, the skilled service of an amiable barber being a perfect example. I urge all gentlemen to acquaint themselves with such an establishment since the convivial glory of the barbershop must be experienced first hand, in the flesh, and without further ado!

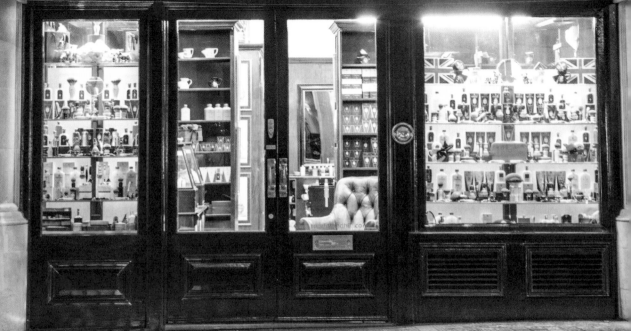

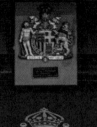

Established 1805

TRUEFITT & HILL

020 7493 2961

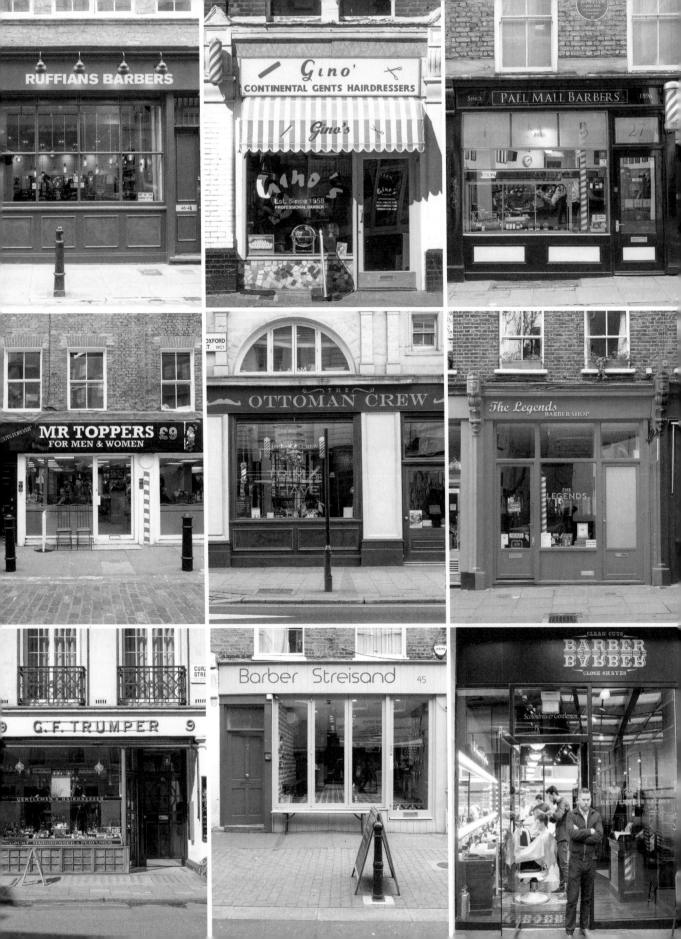

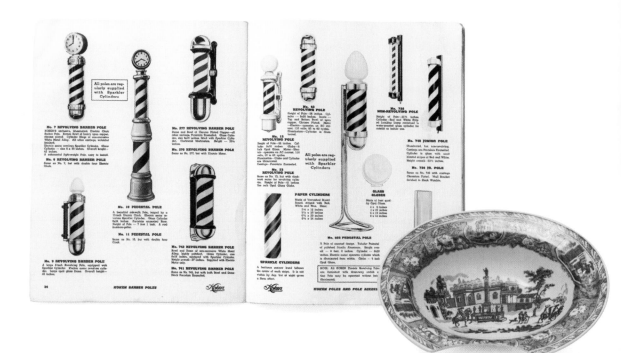

Pole Position

Barber poles from the 1941 Koken catalogue and barbers' bloodletting bowl c. nineteenth century (above). Barbershops of London, variations on a theme (previous pages). ❧

IN THE LAST hundred years the barbershop has had its ups and downs, but it is now an established feature of every main street, and there are many fine examples to be found throughout the world. Although it will always be subject to the vagaries of fashion, the barbershop remains a much-needed retreat from the hustle and bustle of everyday life. Barbers don't just clip men's hair, they get under the skin of the community. From providing refuge for men of color in eras of segregation or for recent immigrants to enjoy familiar humor and news from home, they have in common a place for men of all types to chew the fat, free from judgment.

As we have seen, in medieval times, when barbers doubled as surgeons and dentists, the barber's pole was a sure indicator of the business carried out within. However, following King Henry VIII's amalgamation of barbers and surgeons into the Barber-Surgeons Company in 1540, a statute stipulated that barbers should hang a blue-and-white pole outside their premises, while surgeons should display a red pole with a basin. Later, in America, blue was often added to the red-and-white pole, perhaps as a reflection of the national colors. Other exterior signage has also been used through the centuries, especially as manufacturers began to compete, with companies such as Brylcreem, Jeris, and Wildroot donating tin signs to

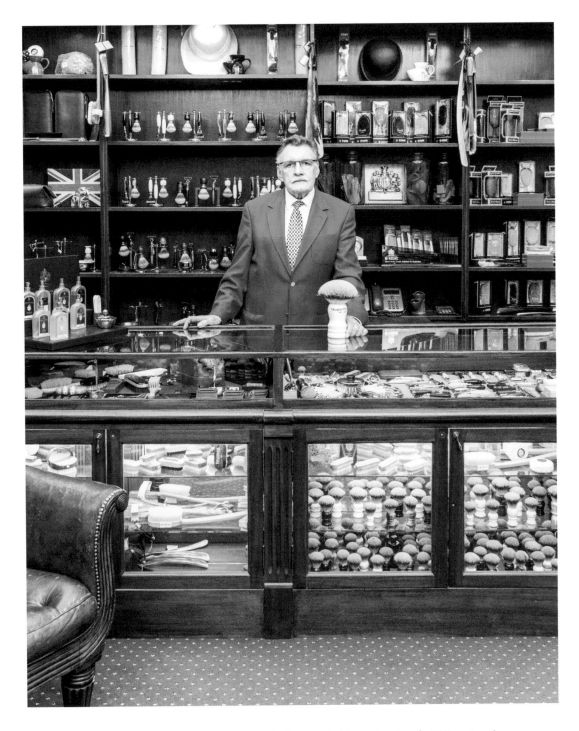

*James Demetrios, a stalwart at Royal Warrant-holding Truefitt & Hill in London
for more than 45 years.*

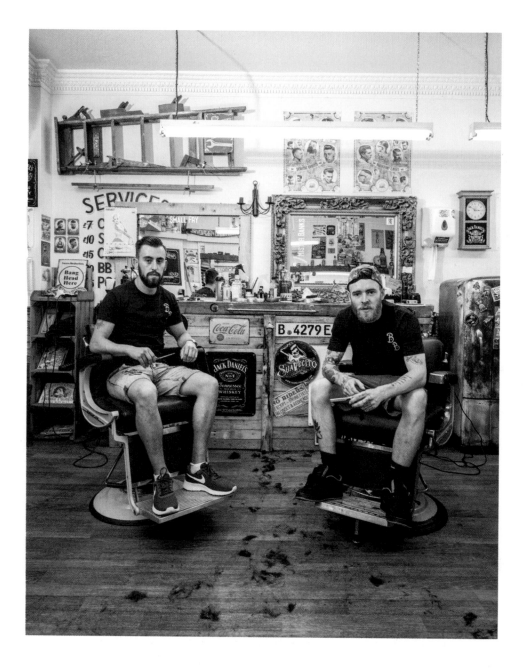

FIXTURES & FITTINGS

Announced by the striped barber's pole, typical furnishings range from time-polished wooden chairs to plush velvet thrones that vie for position before wash basins and chrome-framed mirrors reflecting a reassuring continuity.

The Barber's Chair

EVEN THE SIMPLEST chairs can be things of wonder: they can rotate, lean backward, or adjust their height with the simple press of a lever or a tap of the toe. This bella machina, often glinting with polished chrome and upholstered in beautiful hide, can cost anything up to $4,000, requiring a lot of haircuts and beard trims to pay for them.

Before the mid-nineteenth century, barber chairs resembled ordinary dining chairs. They sometimes had extra long legs for added height and often a fixed-position head rest. The year 1850, however, saw the beginning of a period of innovation, and mechanical chairs specifically made for barbershops began to be produced. Initially, they were in two sections: wooden frames with a padded upholstery seat. The backrest reclined for the customer's comfort and to facilitate the barber's posture. There was an upholstered footstool portion for leg support.

By 1876, manufacturers such as Archer and Berninghaus were producing mechanized chairs. Archer's No. 5 model eliminated the need for a footstool and the No. 9 reclined but also could be raised and lowered manually. Berninghaus patented their Paragon model, a chair that swiveled and could be rotated to "command the advantage of light."

Soon, hydraulics were introduced and one-piece chairs were being manufactured that swivelled 360 degrees and reclined fully. The hydraulic pump enabled the barber to adjust the height of the seat using a foot treadle on the base of the chair. Heavy but stunningly beautiful, boasting intricate carvings and moldings, these chairs were built to last, and did for decades.

Round, cast-iron platform bases began to replace four legs, some coated with wooden veneer to match the upper chair, others painted with black enamel or coated with fired porcelain. These offered enhanced stability. Completely porcelain chairs became the norm as the public became more concerned about cleanliness following epidemics of communicable diseases early in the twentieth century.

Take a Seat

Rattan was often used in warmer climates, allowing air flow and keeping the client cool as the proverbial cucumber (right). ❧

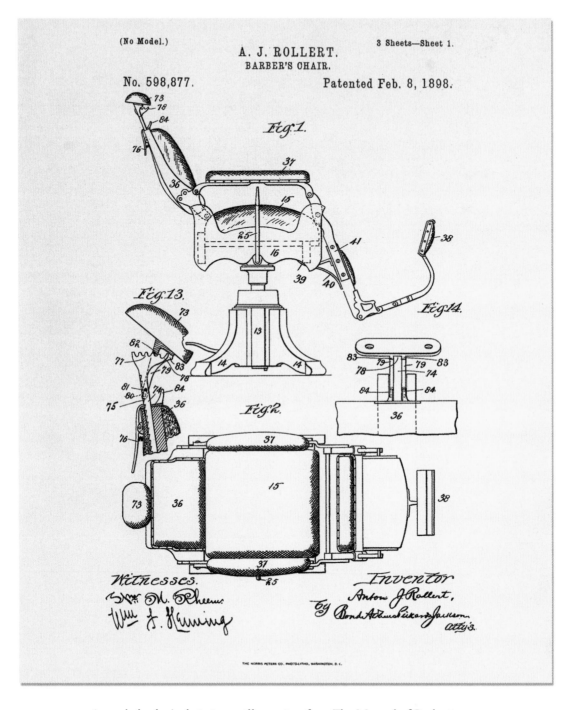

An early barber's chair in an illustration from The Manual of Barbering
by A. B. Moler, 1906.

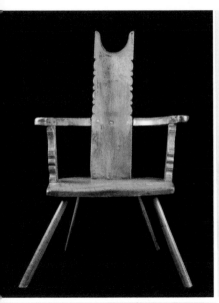
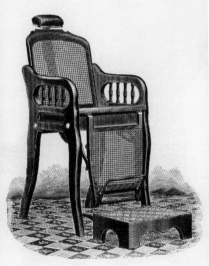
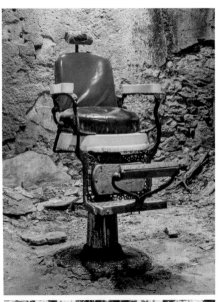
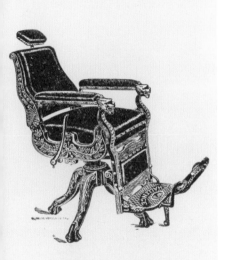
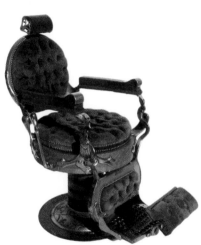
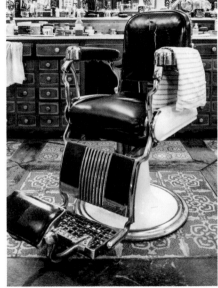
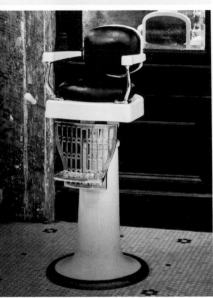
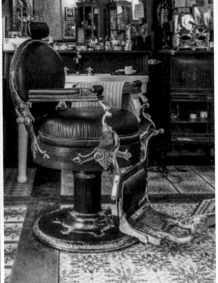
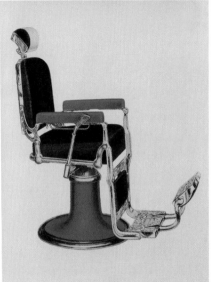

Chairs produced around this time also enjoyed the benefits of improved technology and they lasted indefinitely.

Sadly, by 1950, this striving for perfection was coming to an end, as barber chair manufacturers realised that by producing indestructible chairs they were killing their business. Furthermore, barbershops began to decline in number, and those that existed were opting for cheaper, Japanese-produced chairs.

Nowadays, as the popularity of the barbershop increases, proprietors are seeking, finding, and restoring antique chairs for everyday use, and, as a consequence, barber chairs are now eminently collectible and often sell for many thousands of dollars.

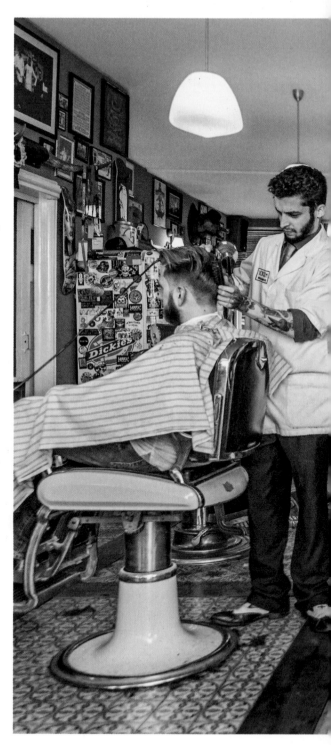

Strictly a Male Preserve
A typical day at Schorem Barbers, Amsterdam. ❧

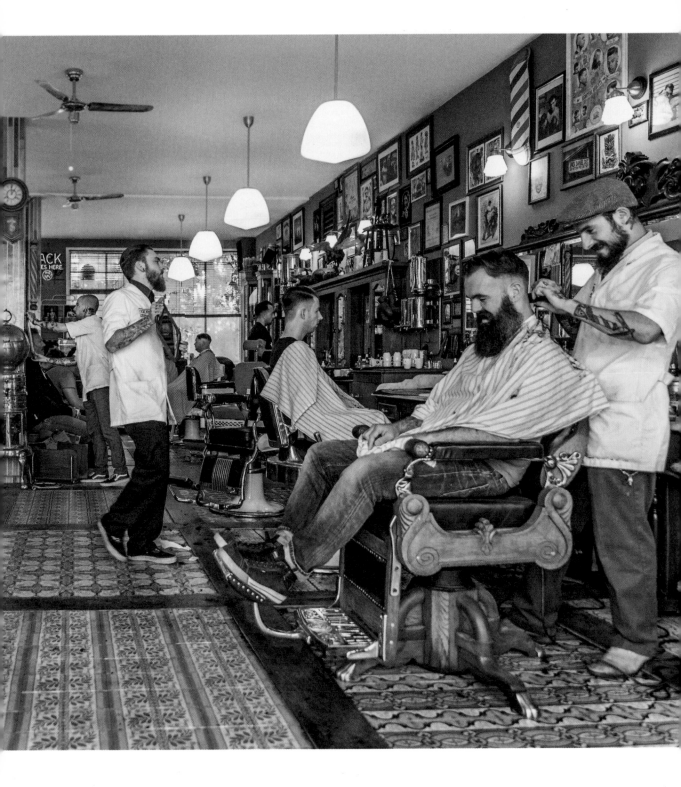

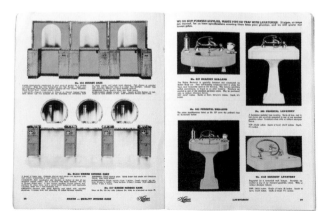

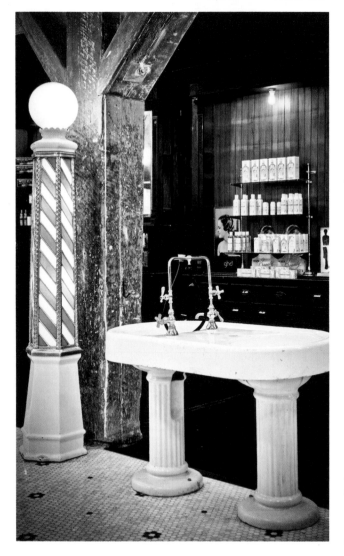

Sinks & Mirrors

SINKS WERE ONCE considered a requirement in every barbershop, firstly to allow barbers to wash their hands, but also to provide water for shaving or for shampooing. In the late Victorian period, barbershop sinks could be elaborate, mounted in cabinets made of walnut, mahogany, or oak with marble bowls, backsplashes, and countertops. Others used French veneers or inlays. By 1900, however, they were being made of white porcelain or coated cast iron, allowing for easier cleaning. Sink bases became less elaborate and more geometric with the advent of the Art Deco style in the 1920s. Thereafter, function won over style, and the sink was simpler and was wall-mounted often into the backbar, the row of mirrors in front of the barber chair.

Before 1900, backbars housing personalized shaving mugs and other essential equipment were often made from elaborately carved wood such as walnut or mahogany, usually very expensive, but an integral and essential part of the shop. This feature became less ornate with the introduction of basins and running water.

As the twentieth century progressed, with the arrival of plastics, everything was white to demonstrate cleanliness. Sterilizers began to appear, and, with the ready availability of electricity, lighting was mounted around the mirrors. With the increased use of spray bottles to spritz the hair and steamers to warm towels for a traditional shave, basins are becoming less common and are no longer considered an essential fitting.

Getting into Hot Water
1941 Koken catalog (above left). Ludlow Blunt in Williamsburg, New York city (below left). Gentleman & Rogues Club, Poole, U.K. (opposite). ❧

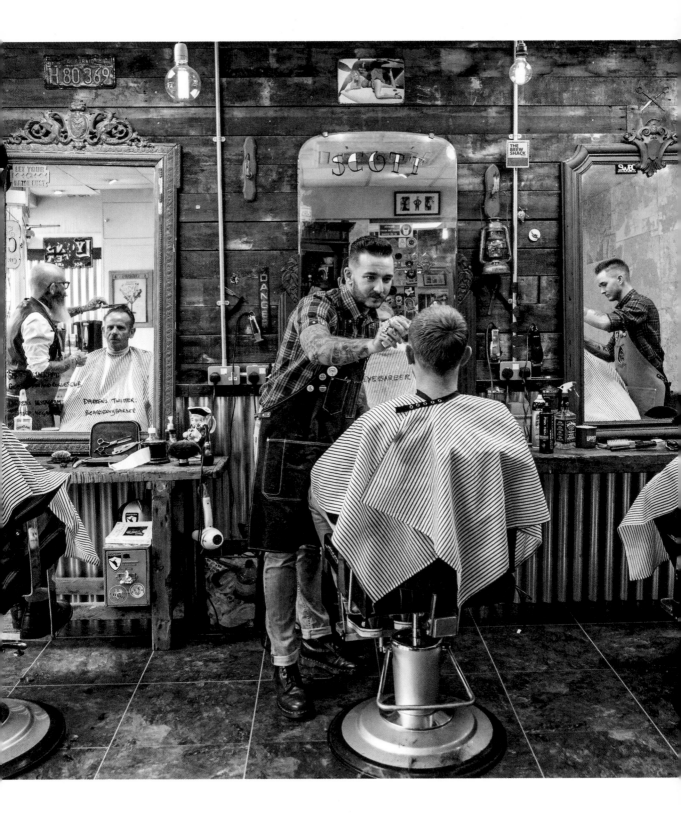

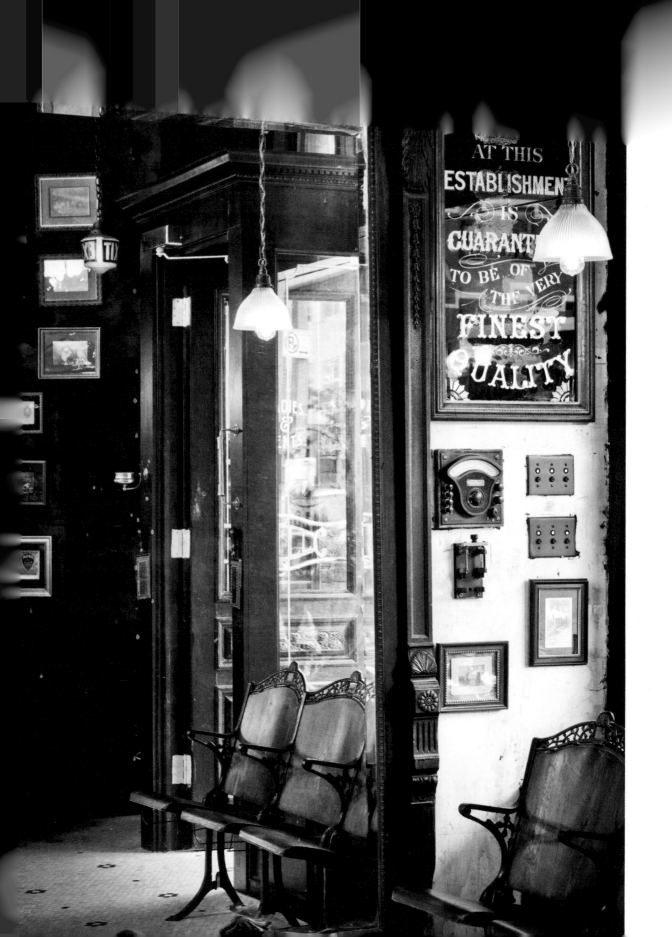

Wall Treatments

THE WALLS OF a traditional barbershop tell a story, an intriguing tapestry consisting of layers of history bearing witness to both the life of the owner and his neighborhood.

These montages of personal effects might illustrate political allegiances, favorite football teams, and feature ads highlighting the everyday stuff of male life from styptic pencils and cheap cologne to beer and condoms. ("Something for the weekend sir?") Collectible tools might hang alongside treasured family photos, with saucy faded pin-ups peeking from behind images of home, since many barbers were originally established by immigrants. There might be dog-eared snaps of villages in Turkey, Italy, Morocco, or Jamaica. There could be murals, old movie posters, neon signs, foreign bank notes, trophies, autographed celebrity photos, polaroids, maps, pages torn from magazines, newspaper cuttings, and religious symbols reflecting both urban and rural cultures across the globe.

The walls of the modern barbershop are likely to be more self conscious, designed with a desired look rather than displaying the accumulation of a life lived. Hip and carefully considered, they still reflect the tastes and idiosyncrasies of the owner. Skull and tattoo imagery is popular, as are ads for drinks with

The Walls Have Years
A barber shop wall reflects the origins and interests of the barber and his clientele, retaining a distinct personality. Ludlow Blunt, Brooklyn, New York (opposite). Angel's Barbershop, Seligman, Arizona (below). ✺

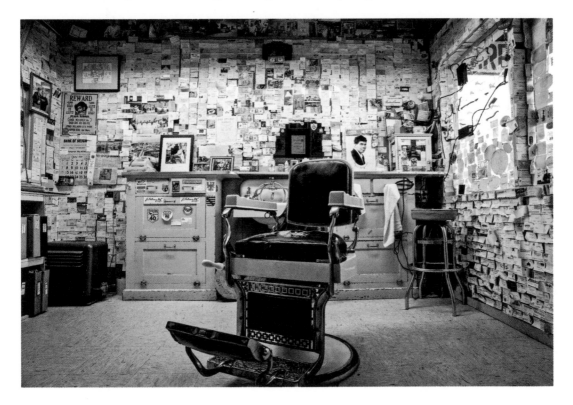

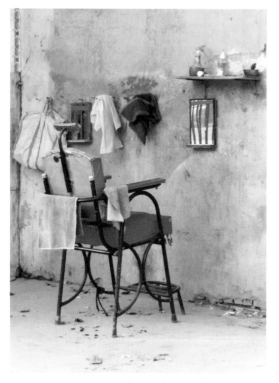

a masculine twist, like Jack Daniel's and Sailor Jerry's, which may well be available to the client.

In traditional and modern establishments alike there are photos of inspirational hairstyles to help the customer articulate his desire. Images of quiffs, flat tops, and DAs still paper the walls of long-standing shops, and current posters of retro homage typify our modern affection for past crowning glories.

Above all, these walls reflect the barbershop as a hub of human interaction, a gathering place for political debate or idle banter, and whether old school or street smart this is still the place a fellow comes to "have his ears lowered."

Framing Faces
Street barber, Kanpur, India (left), Beards 'n' Barnets Barbers, Bedfordshire (bottom), Truefitt & Hill, London (top right), Calgary, Alberta (bottom right). ❧

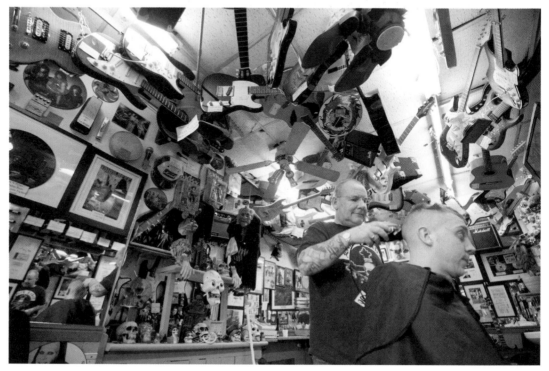

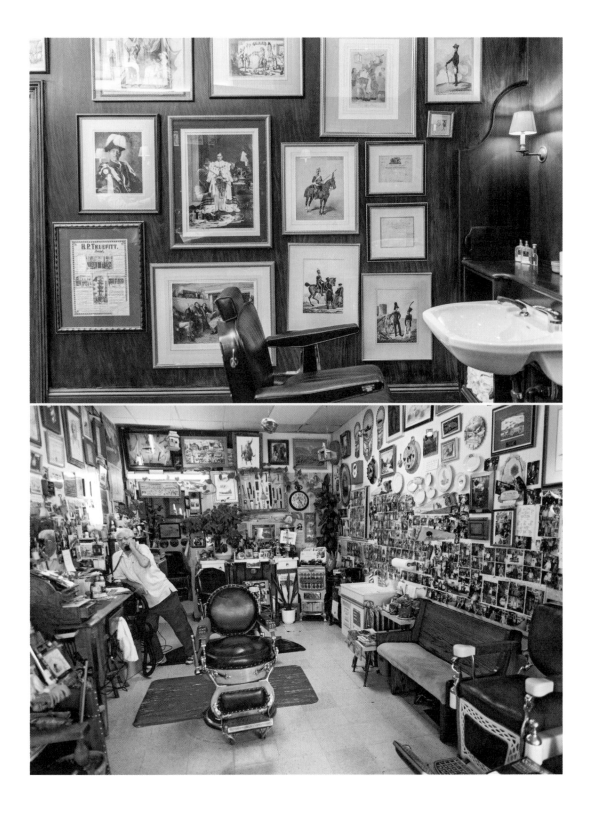

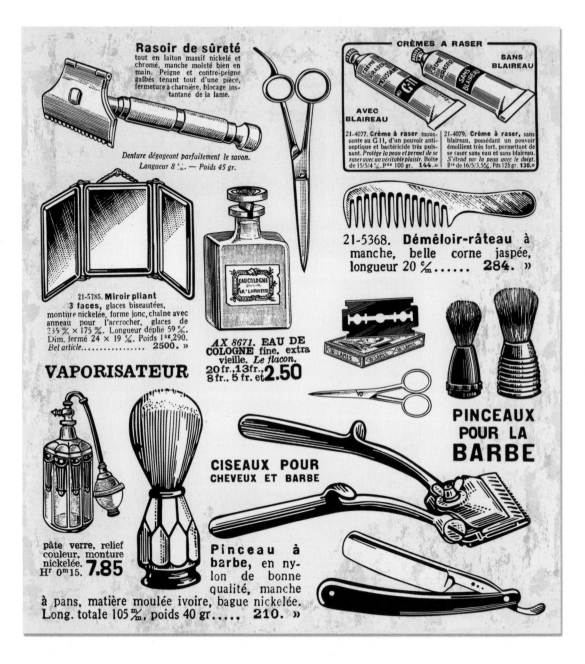

Rasoir de sûreté
tout en laiton massif nickelé et chromé, manche moleté bien en main. Peigne et contre-peigne galbés tenant tout d'une pièce, fermeture à charnière, blocage instantané de la lame.

Denture dégageant parfaitement le savon.
Longueur 8 ℅. — Poids 45 gr.

CRÈMES A RASER

AVEC BLAIREAU

SANS BLAIREAU

21-4077. **Crème à raser** moussante au G II, d'un pouvoir antiseptique et bactéricide très puissant. *Protège la peau et permet de se raser avec un véritable plaisir.* Boîte de 15/5/4 ℅. Pᵈˢ 100 gr.   **144.»**

21-4079. **Crème à raser**, sans blaireau, possédant un pouvoir émollient très fort, permettant de se raser sans eau et sans blaireau. *S'étend sur la peau avec le doigt.* Bᵗᵉ de 16/5/3,5℅. Pds 125 gr.   **130.»**

21-5368. **Démêloir-râteau** à manche, belle corne jaspée, longueur 20 ℅......   **284.** »

21-5785. **Miroir pliant**
3 faces, glaces biseautées, monture nickelée, forme jonc, chaîne avec anneau pour l'accrocher, glaces de 235 ℅ × 175 ℅. Longueur déplié 59 ℅. Dim. fermé 24 × 19 ℅. Poids 1ᵏᵍ,290. *Bel article*...............   **2500.** »

VAPORISATEUR

AX 8671. **EAU DE COLOGNE** fine. extra vieille. *Le flacon.*
20 fr..13 fr.. 8 fr.. 5 fr. et **2.50**

PINCEAUX POUR LA BARBE

CISEAUX POUR CHEVEUX ET BARBE

pâte verre, relief couleur, monture nickelée. Hᵣ 0ᵐ15. **7.85**

Pinceau à barbe, en nylon de bonne qualité, manche à pans, matière moulée ivoire, bague nickelée. Long. totale 105 ℅, poids 40 gr.....   **210.** »

TOOLS & KIT

Scissors, clippers, combs, and brushes, along with the infamous cut-throat razor, have been essential tools of the tonsorial artist's trade for many a century. These classic designs continue to be honed and enhanced, ensuring the modern barber is at the cutting edge.

Scissors & Clippers

ASKING A BARBER about his or her scissors can be a mistake unless you have several hours to spare. This versatile tool can become an obsession. Barber's shears, as they are also known, are significantly sharper than ordinary scissors and usually with an appendage—a finger brace or tang attached to one of the rings through which the finger fits. They are made of stainless steel, with steel from Japan reckoned to be the highest quality. The best will have been hand-forged, as opposed to cast or stamped and as such will have a sharper edge, which will be convex. When both blades of a good pair of hair-cutting scissors are closed, they should touch each other only at the very tip of the blade. This slight bow is so that as they are closed, the built-in tension will allow them to bite and cut the hair cleanly instead of it sliding along the blade.

Barber's scissors come in a variety of sizes, with the smaller ones being especially useful in creating a tailored shape. Longer ones are more effective when a technique such as scissor over comb is used. Texturizing scissors, with one blade having teeth like a comb, are used to thin hair, to create texturizing effects, or to thin and blend layered hair.

Another essential barbering tool are the clippers. Nowadays, of course, they tend to be electric, but manual clippers were once the norm. They were invented in the late 1800s by a Serbian barber, Nikola Bizumic, who became wealthy as a result of his revolutionary invention. They consisted of a pair of sharpened blades that slid sideways when the handles were squeezed, cutting hair close to the scalp. They required frequent lubrication and were very hard on the hands of barbers, who had to use them all day, every day. Early versions

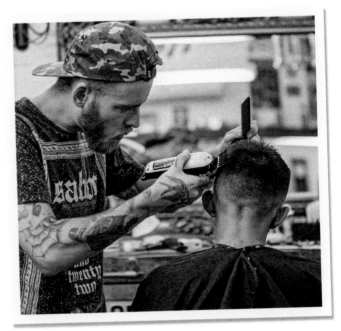

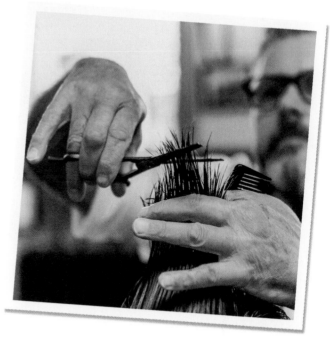

Well Kitted Out

Tools for the tonsorial artists (opposite). Sean Banks of Banks Barbers, Wisbech (top). Robert Lagerman of the New York Barbershop, Rotterdam (bottom). ✳

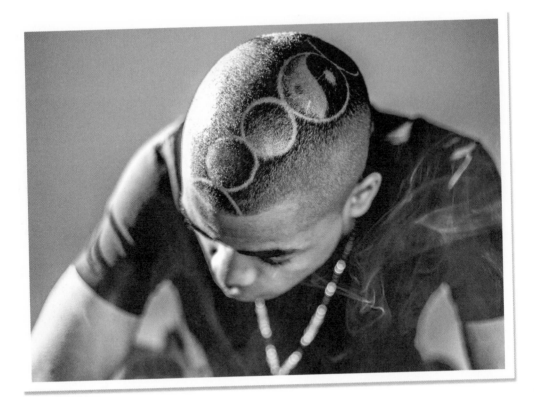

could be uncomfortable for customers, too, as failure to perfectly close the handles could result in painful plucking from the root instead of shearing the hair.

In electric clippers, the blades are driven from side to side by an electric motor. The first pair of clippers powered by electricity was invented by Leo J. Wahl and patented in 1921. Within a year, he had sold thousands of his clippers through his company, the Wahl Clipper Corporation. His business survived his death in 1957 and now makes products for the professional beauty salon and barber trade as well as for consumer personal care and even animal grooming.

Fine Lines
The artistry of modern barbering seen here with perfectly precise patternwork courtesy of Kade Kut, Bedford, U.K. (this page). Tools of the trade (opposite). ❧

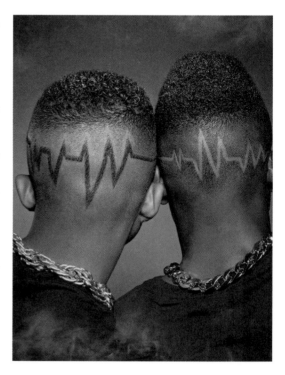

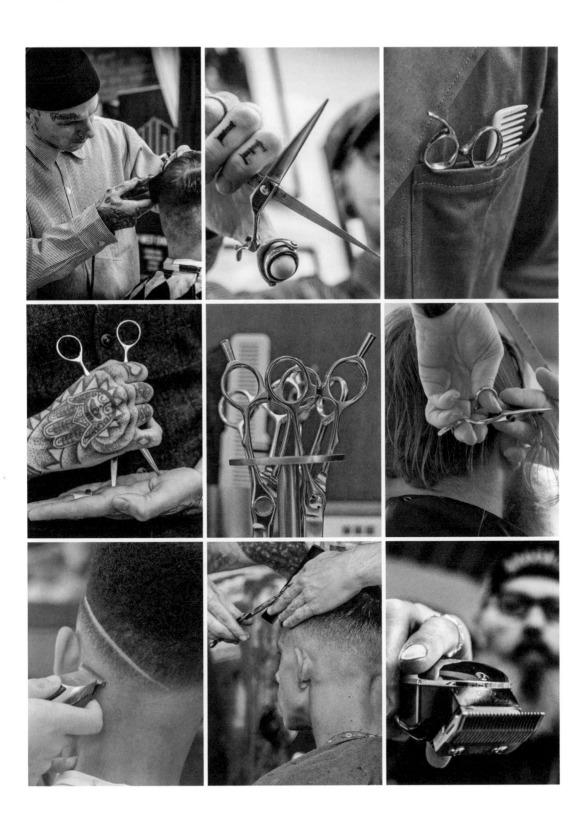

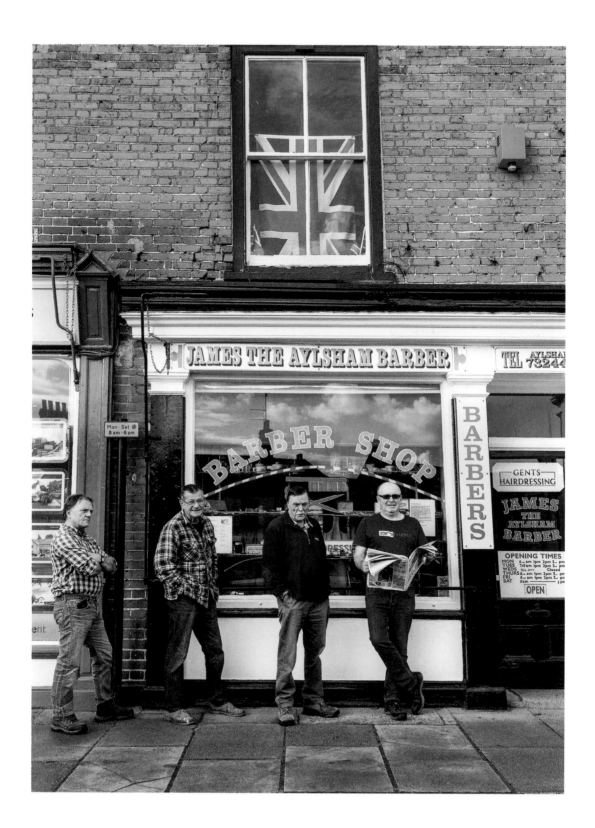

THE LOCAL BARBER'S SHOP

*Found in traditional towns from time immemorial, this is a welcoming place
where time stops and the world is put to rights.*

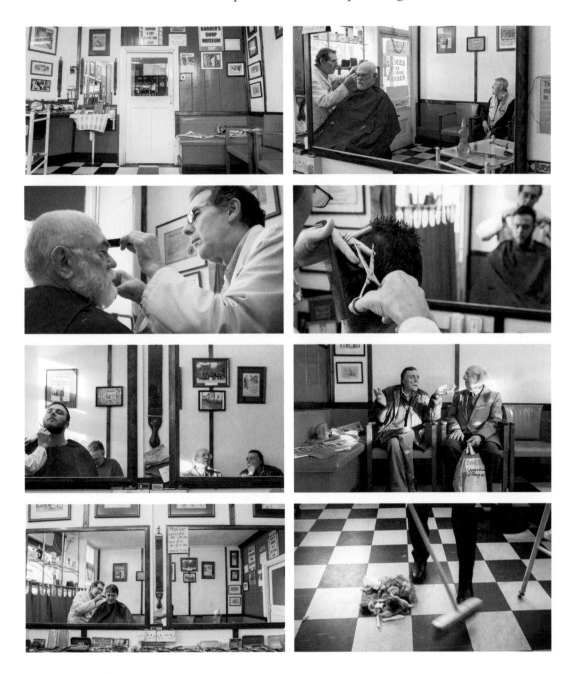

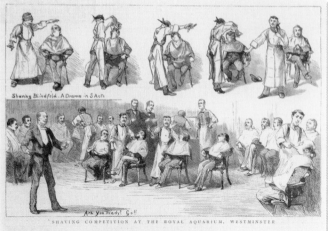

'SHAVING COMPETITION AT THE ROYAL AQUARIUM, WESTMINSTER'

Razor Sharp
The razor strop, often made of leather or canvas, was used in conjunction with an abrasive paste to straighten, hone, and polish the blade. Only the extremely wealthy would own a razor for every day of the week. ✺

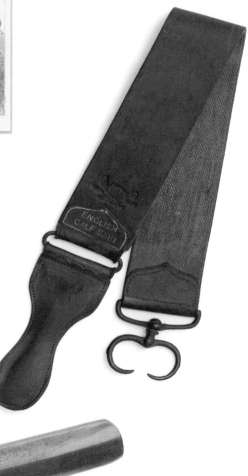

The Cut-Throat Razor

THE NARROW-BLADED folding straight razor has been with us since the first one was manufactured in Sheffield in 1680. Prior to the twentieth century, it was the shaving implement of choice, and in many countries it remained the most common way to shave until the 1950s.

The cut-throat can still be found in its disposable "Shavette" version as used in most barbershops. In fact, the straight razor has a growing number of aficionados who have developed a renewed interest in the art of shaving, with the best blades being made in Solingen, Germany, and in France and Japan.

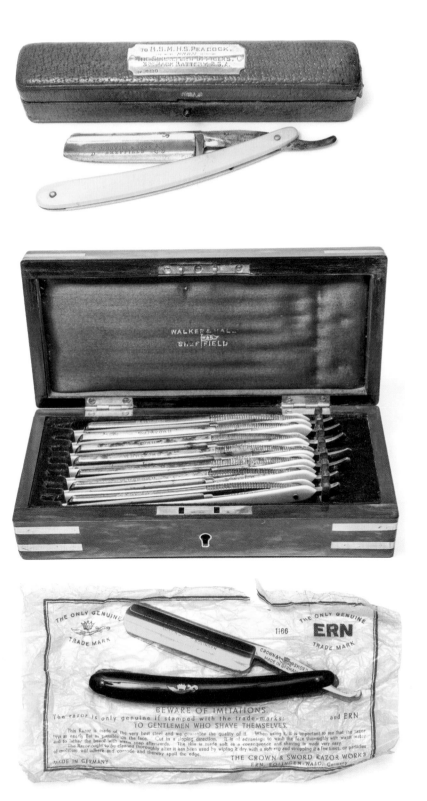

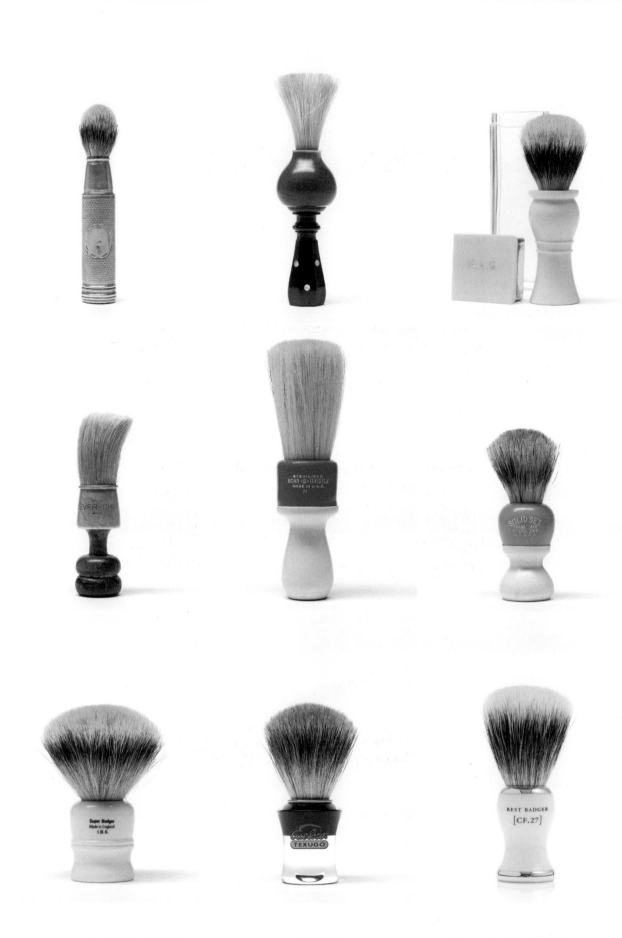

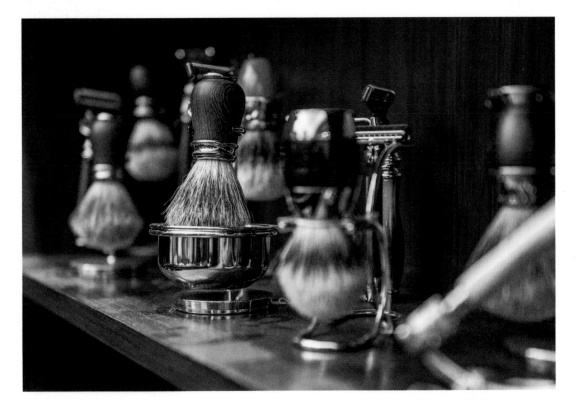

The Shaving Brush

THE SHAVING BRUSH as we know it was invented in France in 1748 and was often made from badger hair, which has led to the French word for shaving brush being *blaireau*, meaning badger. Badger hair was a wise choice; it's hollow, allowing it to retain water and consequently providing a rich lather. (The point of lather, by the way, is disputed. Some say it softens the face prior to shaving, others that it makes the bristles stand up, ready to be shaved off.) Horse hair and boar's hair are also used in shaving brushes; however badger hair is considered to be the best. It is available in four grades—Pure Badger, Best Badger, Super Badger, and, the most expensive and rarest, Silvertip Badger.

In a Lather

A sample of the captain's collection of fine brushes (opposite) with stands being used to allow the brush to drip dry and prolong its life (top). ❊

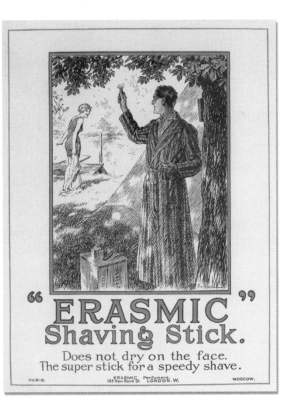

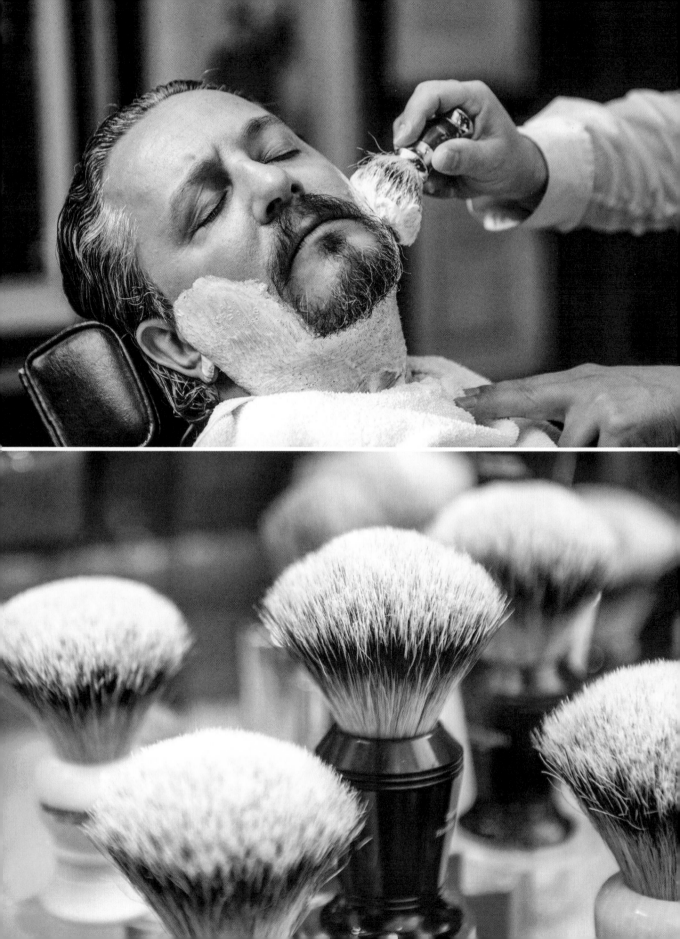

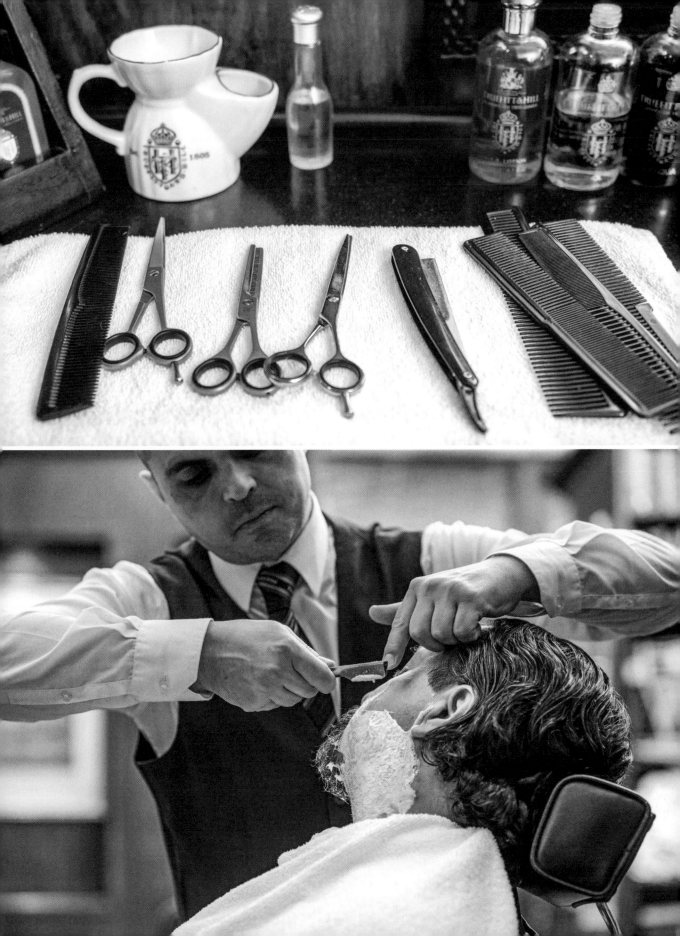

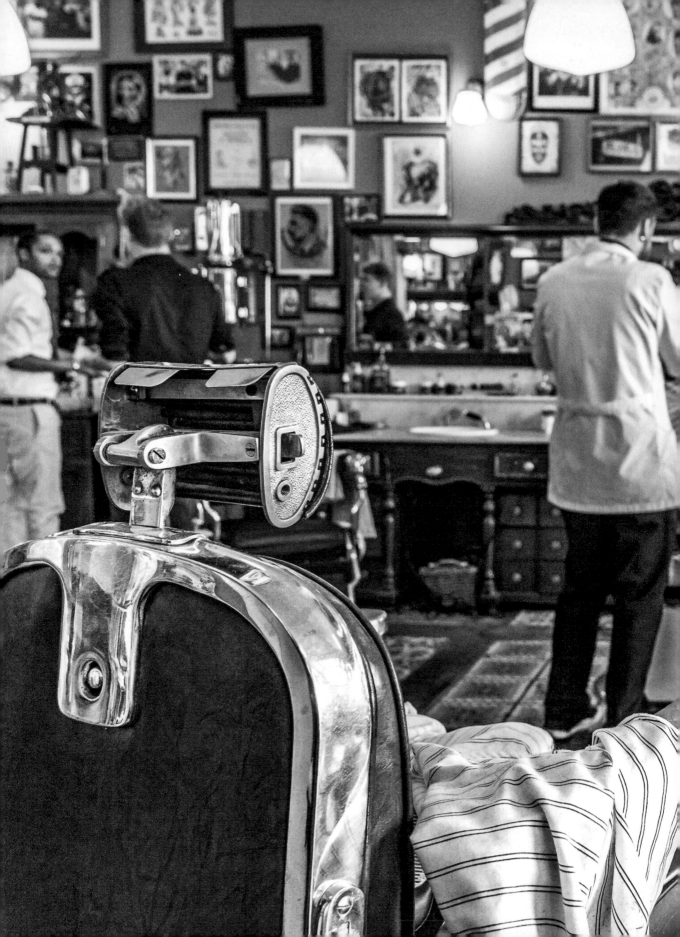

THE BARBERING
EXPERIENCE

FROM THE STREETS OF KOLKATA TO THE SALONS OF
SOHO, BARBERS ARE SKILLED CRAFTSMEN WHO TAKE
PRIDE IN MAKING A GENTLEMAN LOOK DAPPER AND,
MORE IMPORTANTLY, FEEL GOOD ABOUT HIMSELF.

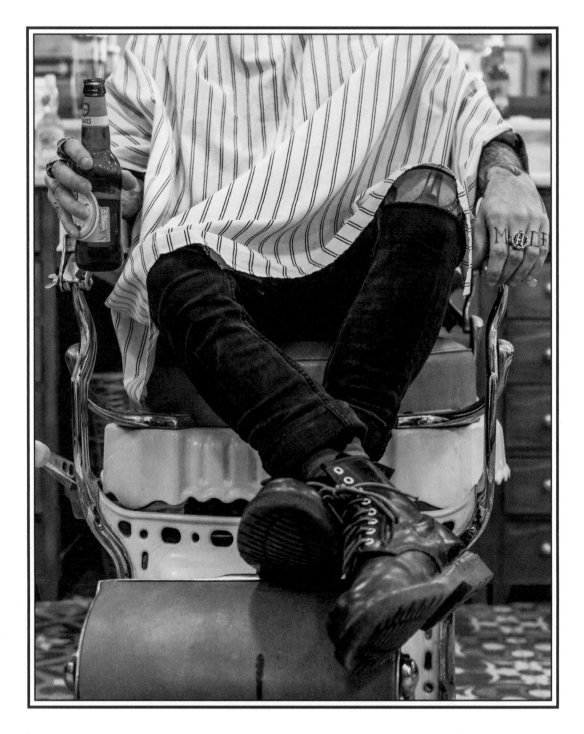

"Something for the weekend, sir?"

I AM HARD PRESSED to think of any other circumstance where a man is warmly invited to sit back and relax while a chap flourishing a cut-throat razor looms large. Yet relax he will, for a visit to one's barber is but time for a true gentleman to unwind in sympathetic society, a chance to converse and to collect himself in congenial masculine company.

ARBERING PRACTICES HAVE deep roots in diverse local and national traditions. The experience, however, while individual and personal, remains universally similar. The relationship with one's barber is extremely special. The person entrusted with your appearance is often a confidante, mentor, and friend. This intimate experience goes far beyond that of a haircut and shave; it can verge on therapy and on occasion approach spiritual discourse. Artists, analysts, and advisers, barbers come to their trade via many routes. The thread they share is a respect for their craft and sensitivity for human contact in all its forms.

People and cultures around the world view hair in many different ways, often imbuing it with magical properties or using it as a signifier of authority or status within a community. Hair is often perceived to be an extension of a person and should not, therefore, be allowed to fall into the wrong hands. Australian aboriginals, for instance, even those living in an urban environment, are extremely careful as to how they dispose of cut hair and take steps against it being used by sorcerers to cast evil spells. This fear of cut hair is also present in some cultures in South Africa, hair being quickly disposed of once shorn. In many other African cultures, hair is thought to be special, even when the person on whose head it has been is dead. In the Congo, hair, along with the nails of a deceased person, is placed in a statuette and kept to maintain the beneficial presence of that person in the home. In Mexico, hair is also believed to possess magical properties, and sorcerers looking to cast spells on people will often first attempt to obtain a lock of their victim's hair to facilitate their sorcery.

In New Zealand, hair has great significance for the Maori culture. In fact, a specific day is traditionally set aside for the cutting of hair, which is accompanied by great ceremony. Those who do the barbering are considered taboo, which means, for instance, that their hands must not touch food. Like the Maori, Japanese sumo wrestlers' hair has ritual significance, and a sumo who is to retire participates in a ceremony—*mage wo kiru*—in which the head of the sumo stable cuts off the sumotori's ritual bun to demonstrate that he has relinquished his position.

Indeed, hair can have significance as a rite of passage or adulthood. A young man of the Masai tribe of Kenya, for instance, participates in a ceremony at the age of 24 in which his mother shaves his head, seated on the same cowhide on which he had been circumcized ten years previously. After several more initiation ceremonies, he is inducted as a junior elder, and at

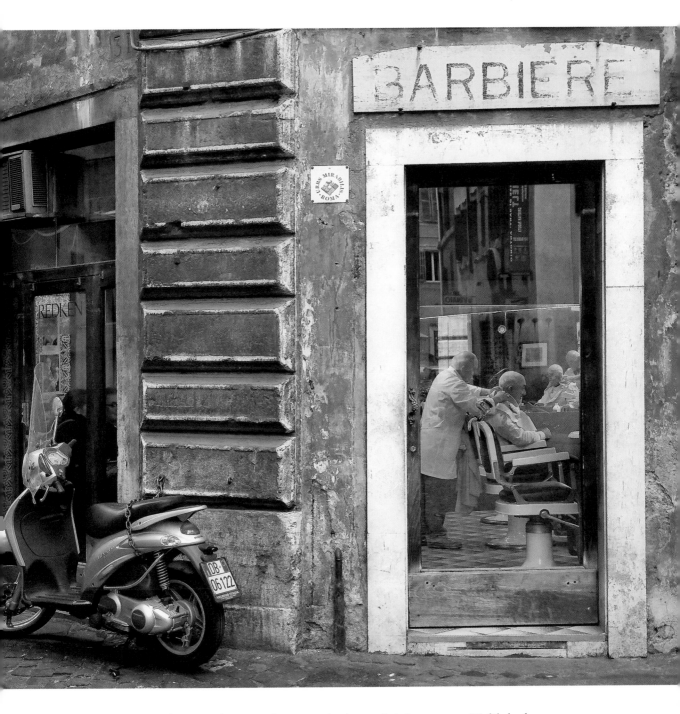

There is a long-standing trust between a barber and their customer. It's likely these elderly gentlemen have shared confidences, passed the time, and grown old together.

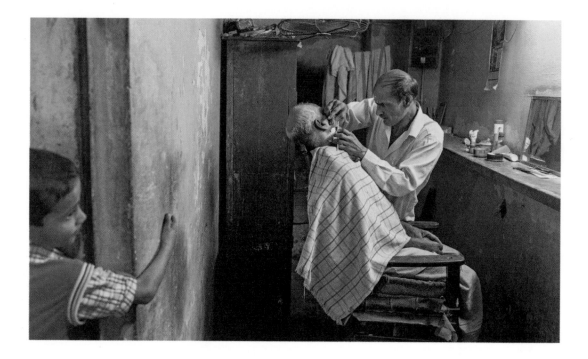

this point his head is shaved again, this time by his wife. Masai men spend hours grooming and even styling each other's hair. Western oils and balms are eschewed for such tonsorial nutrients as ashes, clay, and animal fat.

Meanwhile, for the Yorubas of Western Nigeria and Benin, hair takes on a natural guise. They see it as a bush that provides shelter and protection for the head. In fact, the hairstyle in the past performed a number of roles and functions for the Yorubas. It was a medium of social communication, a signifier of clan. It displayed that its owner had undergone a particular initiation ceremony. It displayed religious beliefs, and, for women, the hairstyle showed their marital status. The Yorubas believe the head to be the seat of the soul, and their phrase for "human beings" can be translated as "humanity, the species that grows hair mainly on the head."

Long hair is traditionally very important to Native Americans and is of religious significance for them. Tradition states that it is to be cut only in the event of the death of a loved one. The cutting of Native Americans' hair, however, developed into a political issue in the late nineteenth and early twentieth centuries. The Federal government insisted that all Native Americans convert to Christianity, and long hair was considered un-Christian. Of course, it could be a desperate thing for a Native American to have to cut his hair. The Hopi tribe of the Southwest, for instance, was entirely dependent for sustenance on the corn it grew, and for the corn to grow rain was needed. Their long hair symbolized rain for them, and to have to cut it off presented them with a terrifying prospect of drought and a subsequent lack of food.

Hair is of great importance to the peoples of the Indian subcontinent where the institution of the barbershop is an ancient one. Barbers usually belong to a hereditary caste or clan—Mangali, Vostaad, Hajjam, Nayee, or Nayi-brahmin. Barbers, who were also surgeons, have also been traditionally used as messengers or go-betweens, and their ability to handle delicate matters means that to this day Indian barbers are often engaged to open the negotiations for an arranged marriage. A barber would often be attached to a village and was paid in kind and given land to work on in return for taking care of the villagers' hair. Initially, barbers would set up under a shady tree, at a market, or at a crossroads, but many villages now have a barbershop—no more than a rickety shed with a mirror and an old wooden chair with an adjustable neck rest for shaving. Among the barbers are several sub-castes, usually regional in origin. For example, Andhra Pradesh is home to two barber communities—the Konda and the Sri.

An Ancient Tradition
Barbers throughout the world plying their trade in streets, sheds, stores, and on railroad station platforms (opposite, below and overleaf). ✶

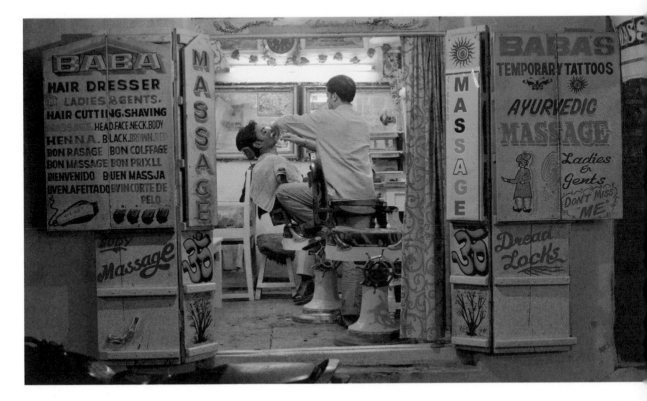

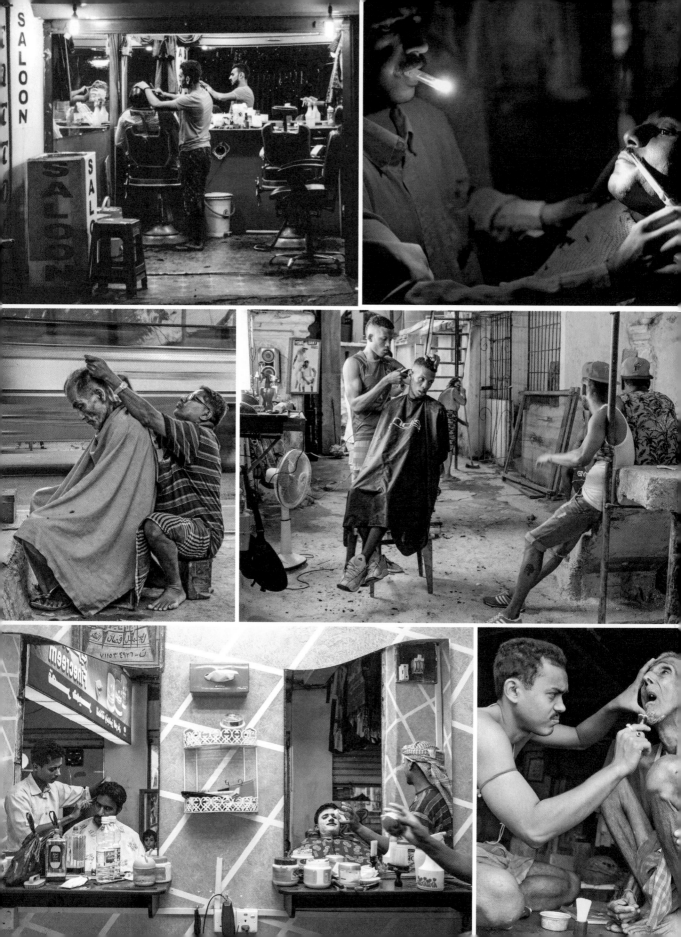

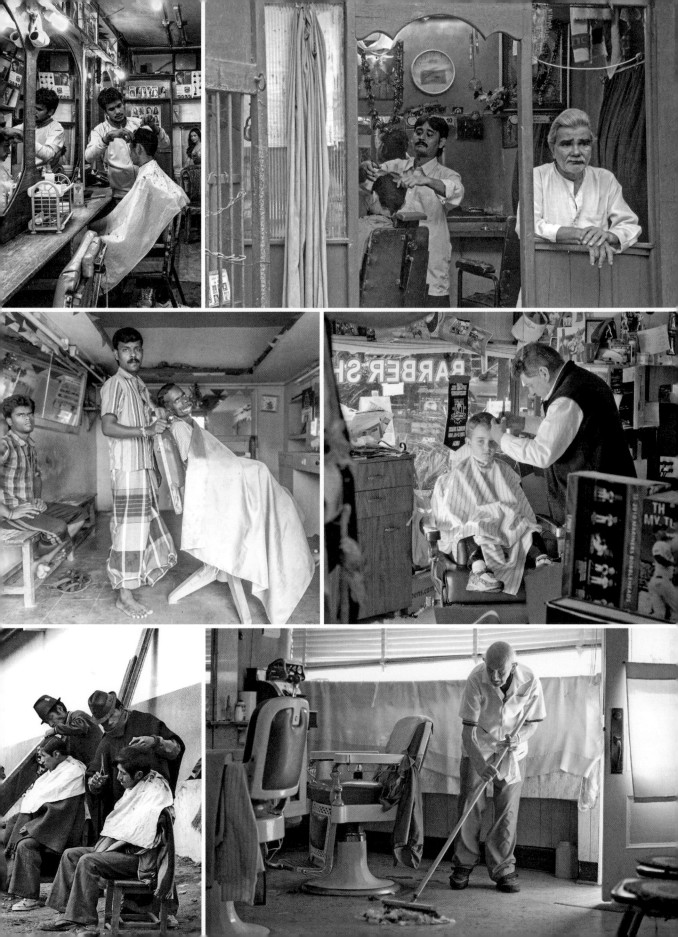

MIGUEL GUTIERREZ
THE NOMAD BARBER

As you are aware, chums, I am not averse to a bit of globe-trotting. That is why I am so impressed with this peripatetic gentleman, who sets up his stool in the far-flung corners of the world. He has traveled to more than 30 countries in 3 years. Well done, that man!

Writer, filmmaker, and entrepreneur, 29-year-old Miguel Gutierrez—aka the Nomad Barber—was born in Liverpool to a Chilean father and a Chinese mother of Burmese ancestry. He has been smitten with barbering since the age of 4 or 5. "As a kid I used to love going to a barbershop run by an old Jewish guy who always had female barbers. I used to love the smell of the talc and the colognes; it wasn't a fancy barbershop, but it still had all these smells." Like many good barbers, he began by cutting his friends' hair at about the age of 14.

"One of my dad's friends owned a few barbershops in Liverpool. He always had a new car, a nice house, and a garden, and I thought maybe that's a good option, better than working out in the cold, getting dirty." Miguel found a job in a barbershop and enrolled on a day-release college course. After working in a number of barbershops in Liverpool and realizing that fancy haircutting was not for him—"I wanted to smash out 30 haircuts an hour in a barbershop where you had proper guys talking about football and stuff"—he began to earn good money. He had always thought travel would be beyond his reach, something only for more privileged people, but when he found himself able to afford a trip to Chile to visit family, he took the plunge. It was the beginning of his love affair with the road. He next spent four months at Camp America before flying to Australia,

> "INDIAN BARBERS ARE SO SPECIAL IN THE WAY THEY USE SCISSORS, A COMB, AND A RAZOR. THEY GENERALLY DON'T USE ELECTRICS. AND THEY STILL GET SUPER-SHARP LINES. MOST PEOPLE SAID THEIR DAD WAS A BARBER, THEIR GRANDAD WAS A BARBER. THERE'S THE CASTE SYSTEM IN INDIA AND THEY ARE BORN INTO THIS ROLE."

From Liverpool with Love
The Nomad Barber following the path of hirsute enlightenment while plying his trade to fund his travels. Seen here clockwise from top: Giant's Causeway in Northern Ireland, Goreme in Turkey Sydney in Australia. ❧

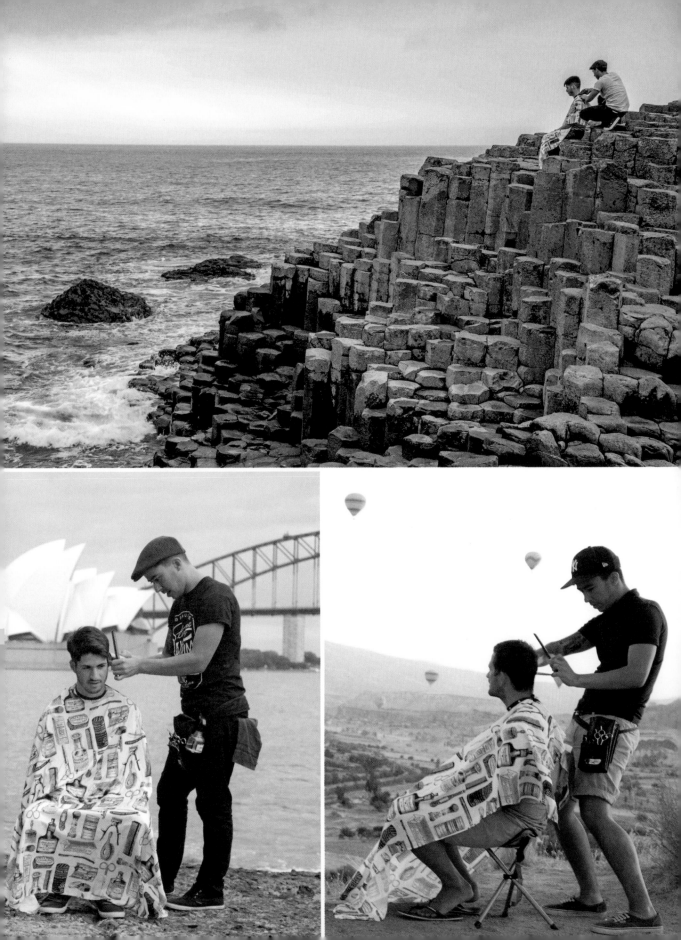

where he found a job in an upmarket hairdresser's by Sydney's Bondi Beach. It was a big step up, and his trial for the job looked like it would be difficult. "I was used to doing short back and sides. I hadn't even picked hair up with my fingers that much to cut it. I just did fast haircuts. Luckily my first customer was an Irish bloke who had a typical Scouse haircut. I got the job!" Ever resourceful, he learned by watching others as they cut.

Returning to London a few years later, he worked in Mayfair and Soho, but the itch for travel would not go away. He found a friend to film him cutting hair in locations around the world, and in June 2013 they set off for Greece, moving on to Turkey, Kurdistan, Dubai, India, Nepal, Hong Kong, Singapore, and Malaysia. "We ended up documenting barbershops around the world. I wanted to know how these barbers lived, where they came from, where they were going, what got them into it."

Miguel is particularly fond of Turkish barbers, with their incredibly close shaves, neck and back massages, and the bizarre art of ear-hair singeing. "They wrap white cotton balls around a metal stick, dip it into an alcohol solution, light it, and tap on the hair very fast. They move so fast it doesn't burn." (See more on the technique of singeing on page 129.) Barbering is a sociable occupation, and in his films barbers talk of their beginnings in the business, their inspiration, and their lives.

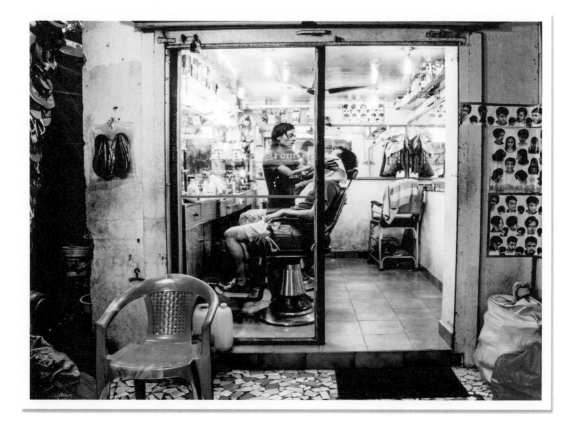

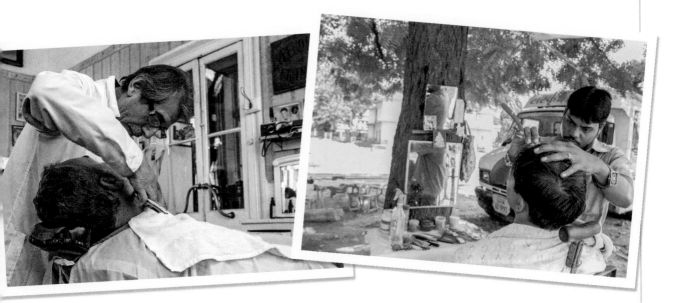

As for the best barbershop, he makes special mention of Antica Barbieria Colla in Milan. Founded in 1904, it has exacting standards; the immaculately groomed barbers keep their unemployed hand behind their backs as they work, in the style of wine waiters in fine restaurants.

Asked what his most challenging haircut was, the Nomad Barber does not opt for a cut in some far-flung corner of the world, but, rather, the very first haircut he did. "I was so cocky when I started working in a barbershop. I would say to the boss, 'Let me cut hair,' and he went to me, 'Go on, then.' I was like 'What?' and he said, 'Go on.' The next customer was a 10-year-old kid, and he was having a number 2 shave all over, and I started doing it, and I was sweating, thinking *Why is this so hard? Why is it not coming off evenly?*" He soon learned.

> "A GOOD BARBER IS SOMEONE WHO'S PASSIONATE, WHO'S DOING IT FOR THE RIGHT REASONS, DOING IT BECAUSE IT MAKES THEM HAPPY, AND THEY'RE GOOD PEOPLE. A BAD BARBER IS JUST THE OPPOSITE, SOMEONE WHO BRINGS A BAD ATTITUDE TO THE SHOP."

Of course, there are many approaches to cutting hair and debate about whether it is an art or just a technique. Miguel has firm views on the subject: "It's not an art. If you're working in a shop, just doing haircuts, it's a craft, a trade. You're doing things repetitively. Maybe if you're a creative hairdresser or a barber doing shows or cutting hair for photo shoots, that's where you can say you're more of an artist."

He may have visited 30 countries, but for the Nomad Barber the journey has just begun.

The Journey Continues
Goa (opposite), Chile (above left), Basava Raj, a street barber from Hampi, India (above right). While Miguel continues to take the road less traveled, the Captain awaits further updates with anticipation. ❧

DARREN HAYWARD OF GENTLEMAN & ROGUES
A COMPASSIONATE MAN

Luxuriantly bearded and often bowler-hatted, Darren Hayward is a deep thinker, yogi, and proud vegan. Convinced everyone has a destiny, however late in life one might find the path, he is a barber with a sense of the spiritual and a proactive social conscience.

Darren Hayward was born to be a barber. When he and his five brothers and sisters played as children, he was always a barber, the tools of his trade the bathroom mirror, a couple of combs, and a large tub of cheap gel from the local supermarket. Later he would watch the hairdresser who came to the house to cut his mother's hair. "That's not a bad way to earn a living," he thought to himself at the time.

He left school at 16 to take up an apprenticeship with a hair salon in his hometown, Poole in Dorset. Like every other hairdressing novice, first he just swept the floor and washed hair. "By the way, I was told you don't call it washing; you call it shampooing. You wash your clothes, you shampoo your hair." It was four or five months before he was allowed near a pair of scissors, his first nervous haircut being inflicted on a girlfriend. "She had a bob ... and went out with a really short bob," he laughs.

Leaving that job, he opened a ladies' salon above another shop, slogging away on his own seven days a week before borrowing £6,000 at the age of 24 and opening a proper salon in Purewell, near Christchurch. By the age of 30 he had six people working for him but was itching to move into barbering, for the camaraderie that he was unable to find working with only female colleagues. After a stint in another salon, he decided to open a barbershop. "I'm a fan of *Boardwalk Empire* and *Peaky Blinders*, and I wanted that retro feel. The metrosexual male had his time. Guys still want to be guys, and the unisex salon wasn't giving them that environment."

As a man who has worked on both sides of the fence, Darren is clear about the issue of

> "BEFORE YOU PICK UP A PAIR OF SCISSORS OR A COMB, YOU HAVE TO HAVE A PICTURE IN YOUR MIND OF HOW THAT PERSON'S GOING TO LOOK. IF YOU'RE IN BARBERING OR HAIRDRESSING, YOU'RE A VISUAL CREATURE. FOR INSTANCE, YOU LEARN HOW TO DO IT BY WATCHING. IT'S ALL ABOUT SHAPE. SHAPE OF THE FACE, SHAPE OF THE HAIR. YOU'RE SCULPTING HAIR."

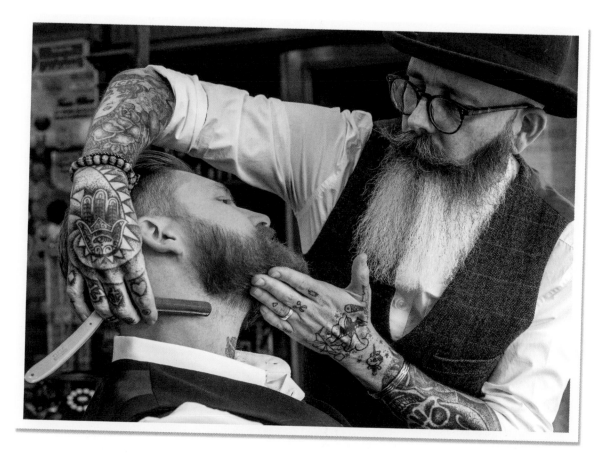

hairdressing versus barbering. "Hairdressing is an art; barbering is a craft. Hairdressers have a much wider variety of colors and styles to work with. Men don't. Regardless of what any other barber will tell you, barbers do the same sort of haircut but in different variations of length. It's the way you dress it out sometimes. So we are craftsmen, and we do a job. You do it over and over again. You nail it. You get it down. It's precision work. That's the difference for me."

Barbers often seem to be visual people, with the ability to see the end result when they start a cut, and Darren Hayward is no different. Communication is key. "When I do a

consultation, I always ask the customer what he does for a living and what his hobbies are. That gives me a good rounded impression of him, and I look at his clothes. What we wear is a way of telling people who we are."

In terms of style, Darren is pretty focused. "We don't cut right up to the crown for instance. We cut to the O-bone at the back. We cut to the shape of the head. A lot of the quick in-and-out barbershops will clip as high as possible. Using scissors takes more time. Clipping right to the top means you spend less time blending with your scissors. We would encourage a customer to have his hair cut to the shape of his head."

Mystic Method
The Hand of Fatima (Arabic) or, depending on your persuasion, the Hand of Miriam (Hebrew), as seen here on Darren's steady hand, invokes protection from the evil eye. ✺

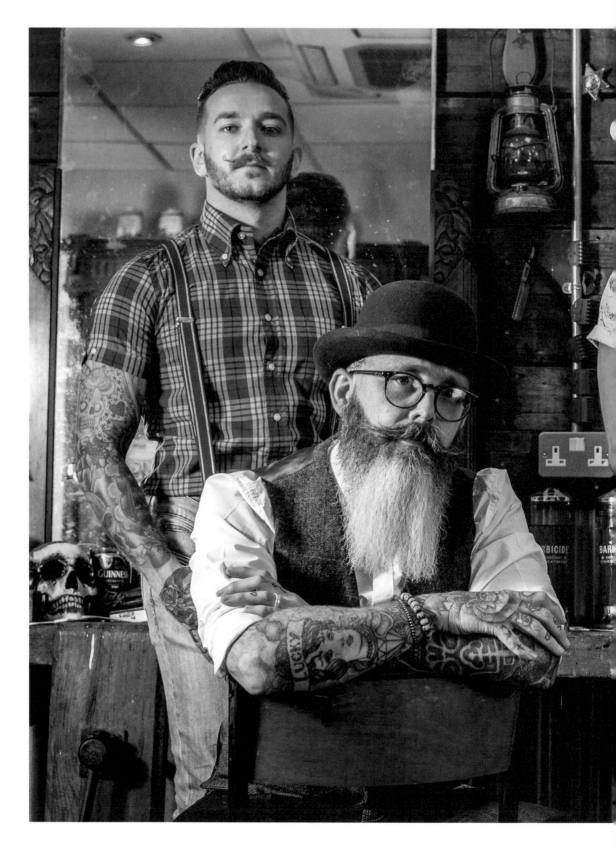

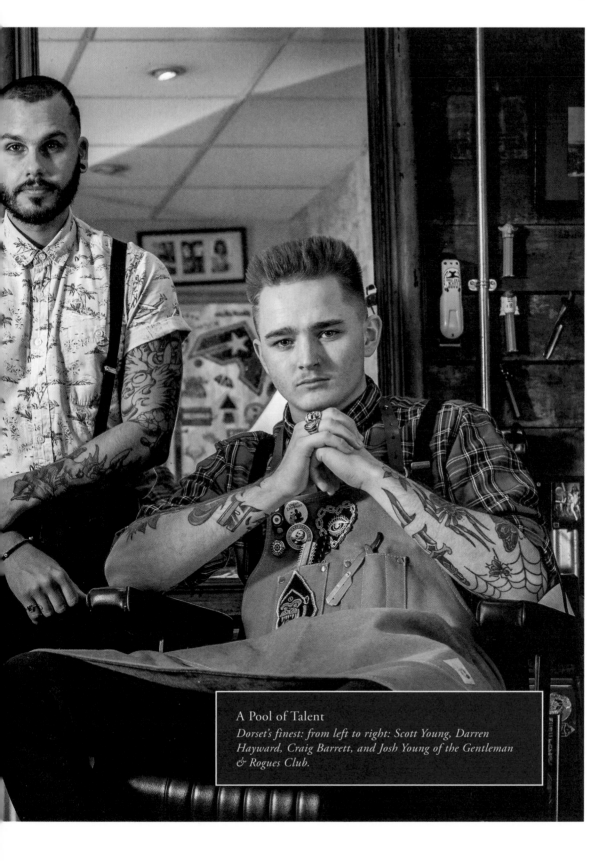

A Pool of Talent

Dorset's finest: from left to right: Scott Young, Darren Hayward, Craig Barrett, and Josh Young of the Gentleman & Rogues Club.

DANI LEWIS OF JOHNNY'S CHOP SHOP
AN INSTINCTIVE APPROACH

Dani Lewis, also known as Toastie Styles, is an excellent barber who knows exactly what she's doing. She admits to being a perfectionist, but it is that relentless drive that makes her work outstanding.

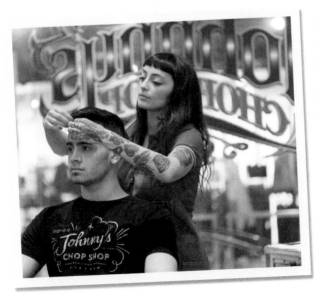

Dani's start is a familiar story: "When I was about 13, I used to do my friends' hair, coloring it and cutting it. I've always been passionate about hair, like I was born to be a barber." But barbering's gain may be art's loss. Dani has an artistic father, and his creative sensibility passed on to her. Perhaps her ability to visualize has proven useful in her development as one of the country's best barbers. "I would draw what I saw in my head, and that's why I think I'm a good hairdresser—what I see I can create. I'll look at someone's hair, and I'll see exactly what I'm going to do. That's what I like about it."

Aged 17, Dani went to hairdressing college, but the learning process was difficult, especially as haircutting to her is instinctive. "I just used to grab a pair of scissors and cut someone's hair, and even if it was wrong it looked good! To me it felt like it was just common sense." After college, she worked in women's hairdressing for a while but never felt at home among the perms and the bobs. The world of the barbershop is a much better environment for her, but it took her a while to find the right one. After various stints in London she spotted Johnny's Chop Shop. "It looked amazing. Checkered floor, really retro, and I thought *That's where I want to work*." She joined them after a few months and has not looked back since.

She brings a strong philosophy to her work. "I think I've done a good job when the haircut looks perfect and the client can style it himself and is happy with it. It needs to be easy for him. It needs to suit his face, it needs to suit his head shape. Everyone thinks it's just a haircut, but there's so much more to it."

NATALIE ANDERSON OF BEARDSGAARD BARBERS
VALHALLA FOR THE HIRSUTE

Good barbers are damned hard to find, especially in out of the way corners like Batavia, Illinois, but Beardsgaard will lavish love and give attention to your hair and beard.

Natalie Anderson is another barber who wanted to be an artist. "It seems to me," she says, "that most barbers can draw. It just seems to be a thing." Perhaps it is a matter of visualization. They have a lot of beards in Batavia, and, as something of a beard specialist, she spends her days doing quick trims, clean-ups, and "beard overhauls." The latter involves a fairly rigorous treatment of deep conditioning, facial hair design, and perhaps even Beardsgaard's legendary "beard blowout," a workout for the beard using a thermal hairbrush and a hairdryer on high heat and low speed. The beard is brushed vigorously upwards to loosen tangles with the dryer blowing hot air on it to make it manageable. It is then brushed down and tamed once more. The result is an exquisitely groomed beard.

Natalie's journey to Batavia began ten years ago when she left her native Chicago for Montreal. She was in Canada on a student visa. This meant, of course, that she had to study something, and, as she had always cut her own hair, she decided to enroll at hairdressing school. The

first shave she undertook with a cut-throat razor was "terrifying," but the client came through the ordeal with his features intact, and a legend was born. A more recent encounter, with Schorem's Bertus and Leen, has confirmed her appointment as a Scum Ambassador extraordinaire.

Natalie describes the Beardsgaard shop—owned with her husband, Tyler—as "nordic and nerdy." And that name—Beardsgaard? They made it up in an effort to come up with a name for a place to which Vikings might go in order to enjoy the rigors of one of their beard blowouts.

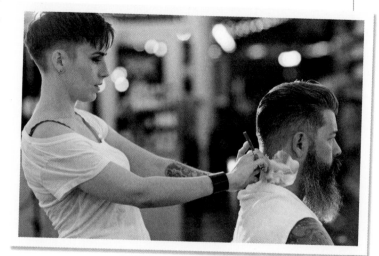

JOSH COOMBES
LIFE-CHANGING HAIR CARE

Josh Coombes, a young hairdresser from Exeter, has created #DoSomethingForNothing to record what he does on city streets, giving haircuts to the homeless.

"I think it was about bringing it down to one person." Josh Coombes is explaining his work. He is talking about a trip he made to Athens with the help of RefuAid to cut the hair of refugees who had arrived from North Africa and the Middle East. "That's what runs through this. When you talk to these people and you look them in their eyes, or someone's handing you this beautiful two-year-old girl so you can cut her hair, you think there's no reason that a mother and father would put their children through this unlessit wasn't hell back home."

This notion of "just one person" is a recurring riff for Josh Coombes. He encourages others to do something, no matter how small, to make people feel they belong. He tells a story of one recent encounter that is fairly typical of what he experiences on a daily basis: "I met somebody today. He's very much looking to get back into work. He's wondering how he can get his life back because he's not in a good place. I could really see that transition from

> "IT'S ABOUT BRINGING PEOPLE WHO FEEL INVISIBLE IN SOCIETY BACK INTO THE LIGHT AND REBUILDING THEIR SELF-ESTEEM. IT'S ALL ABOUT BRINGING IT DOWN TO ONE PERSON AND CONNECTING."

when I first met him when he was so down on his luck and feeling that everything was against him. While I was cutting his hair there were all these other people interacting with him, because people see what I'm doing and stop, wondering what's going on. I always make sure I introduce them to the person whose hair I'm cutting. At the end of the day, I could tell that he was different. Of course, it might be temporary, but he was a different person, his shoulders were straight, he seemed more confident. I think he just felt part of society again."

Josh did not come to hairdressing until fairly late, following a spell after college touring in a punk band. He worked long hours to get through his training and honed what he had learned in a salon. He thought deeply about what he was doing. "I quite soon realized how important that interaction is with the person in the chair in front of you. Homelessness has always been a big issue to me, and it was really simple to begin with. I just went out and cut a couple of people's hair in the city. I got in touch with my friend who's a photographer. When he started taking photos and we started putting them on Instagram, that's when there was a bit of a buzz. It was really strong imagery—people could understand the human being behind the photo. And this is very much what it is about, humanizing the issue. When you bring it down to one person and say that this is someone, this is their story, that's what people can really relate to. The haircut facilitates it. Sometimes it results in a big transformation. Sometimes it's something small. But it's all about people's lives and their stories. People relate to it in a big way on social media. But #DoSomethingForNothing isn't just about homeless people. It's really about showing compassion for anybody who might be a bit hard up. Lots of other people are now using it, and it's not just hairdressing. It can be simple stuff like helping an old person with their shopping or having lunch with them. It's not about whether they have a skill, it's about feeling empowered to do something."

Gentlemen of the Road
In many cities across the world, barbers like Josh give of their free time, helping revive self-esteem in those who have fallen on hard times. ❧

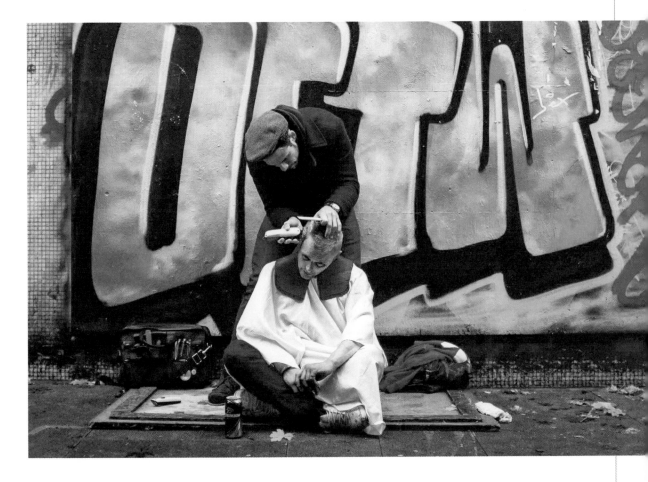

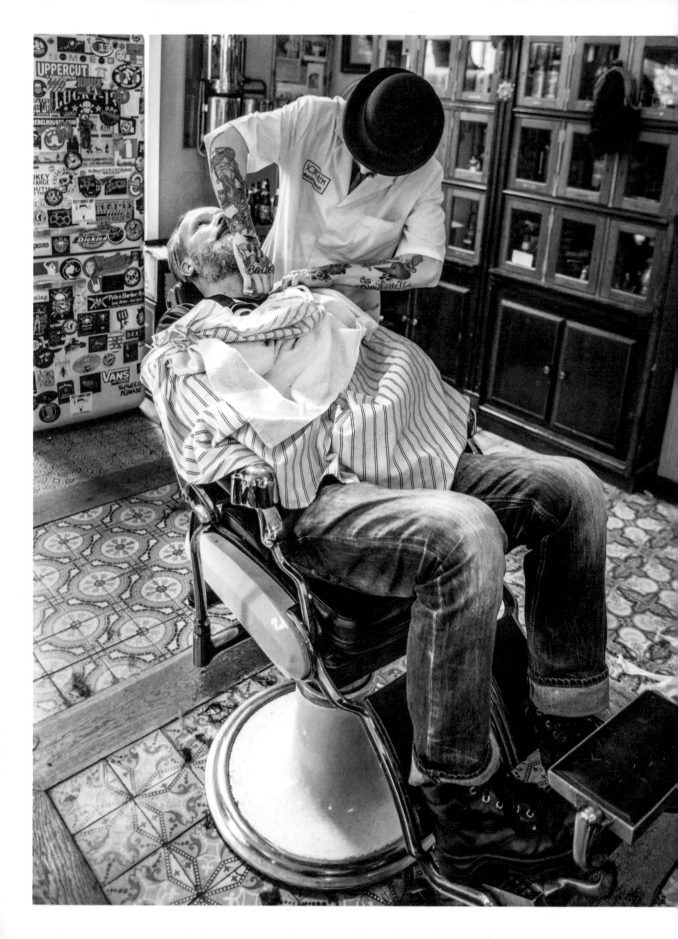

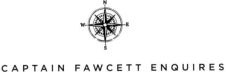

SCHOREM
THE SCUMBAG BARBERS OF ROTTERDAM

I've been in the company of some rum fellows in my time, but these chaps take the ship's biscuit. Although they're from the darker side and sport more tattoos than a Nantucket whaler, they certainly know how to cut a chap's hair and sculpt his beard.

It was a strange business plan—a barbershop offering just four styles of haircut and calling itself Schorem, Dutch for "scumbag." That was six years ago, and, although Bertus and Leen, the shop's founders, are loathe to make comparisons, it is now one of the best barbershops in the world. Every morning when they turn up for work, there is a line of at least twenty men hailing from all around the world in search of one of their classic haircuts. "We wanted to do haircuts that have proven themselves over the decades and will never go out of fashion. Those are the basis of every haircut there is."

As seems quite common among barbers, they began young. Bertus was about fourteen when he started cutting hair. "I wasn't really doing well at school. I just wanted to smoke weed and ride my skateboard. So, I was with a couple of friends, and one of the guys goes, 'Hey, man, I want a mohawk.' My dad had clippers and that was pretty much my first haircut. By the way, I totally screwed it up!" Word spread, and his friends would bring in album covers from which he would copy the hairstyles.

Seeing where his interests lay, his mother sent him to beauty school, but learning how to perm hair was not his thing. So, aged sixteen, he found a job in a barber's and began to learn his trade. "I really, really loved it. I mean, I don't like it when hairdressers go, 'Oh, it's my life!' but I have to be honest, it kind of was. I wanted to know everything there was to know about it. I wasn't good at anything, really. But hair I understood, and I've always loved the margins of society. So, I loved the whole punk thing, and haircuts were just a part of it."

Bertus's musings on cutting hair are fascinating: "The weird thing about doing haircuts is it's really not that hard to learn, but it takes a lifetime to master it. Every time you think you know it you find out you don't know anything. It's a bit of math, and it's a bit of being creative, but everybody can learn how to cut hair. You have a tool in the right hand that cuts the hair off—whether it's a clipper or a pair of scissors—but it's the left hand that matters. How you hold the comb, that's going to make the haircut. The right hand isn't really that

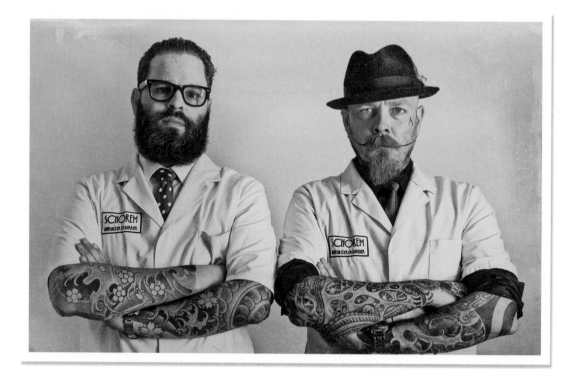

important, but that's all stuff you find out later. The head is round—so if you cut a straight line here, you should think about what is going to happen. You should be able to say, well that is what is going to happen because it's math, it's round, and it's straight lines. It's super-interesting. I've been doing it 27 years, and only now do I have the feeling that I'm kind of getting the hang of it."

Does such a limited palette not get boring? Bertus insists that, of course, every head is different, and "You are an artist, and you have to re-invent yourself every 45 minutes ... What I love is that you cannot lie with your hands. You can lie with your mouth, and you can lie with your eyes—people are really good at it—but your hands really show it. Whether you build a bike or you work with wood—any product in the world—you can stand next to it, and you can see exactly what's happening, and that's beautiful. When you look at it, you're never done learning. A carpenter will make chairs and tables his whole life, and they get more and more beautiful the older he gets because he learns how to read the wood and how to use his tools, and it gets better and better, but in the end it's still a table and chair. It will never get boring."

The Scumbag Barbers' recruitment policy is unconventional. They hire men living on the streets and even ex-convicts. "We get guys from the street who have absolutely no idea about hair. But it's a craftsman's thing. You will have

Lardy di Dah!
Leen and Bertus really need no introduction: suffice to say they're scum of the earth. Rarely in Rotterdam, they appear to be on a constant world tour spreading the word and recruiting the next generation of Scum Ambassadors. ✦

your pupils standing, watching, and you can see the penny drop. They start with a shave, and the first time they do a perfect shave you can see the pride. So many people have looked down upon them for years. Barbering is a thing from the street. It's not arty-farty. Guys need a haircut."

In a recent newspaper interview, the Scumbags summed up their philosophy: "What we do is not fashion; we do style. We're scumbags. But decent scumbags."

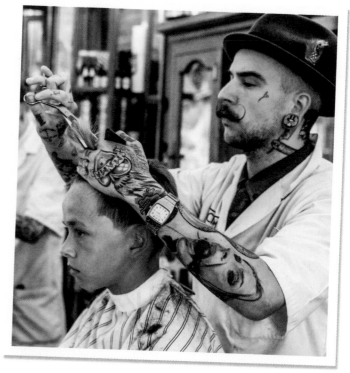

In Safe Hands
Bobbie Bones styles the hair of a new generation (right). Bertus applying the finishing touch to a client (below). ✣

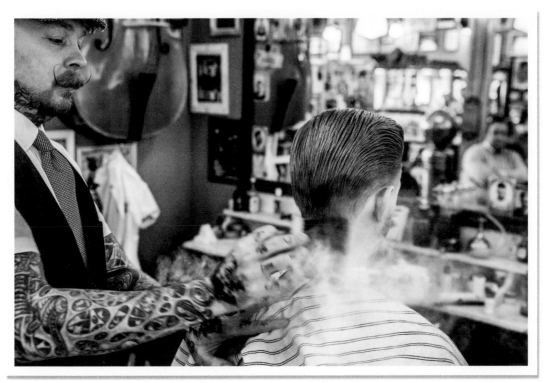

SID SOTTUNG
BARBER & EDUCATOR

Barbering has been Sid Sottung's salvation. During a dark period, he gambled on a notion, and it turned his life around. Always a dedicated teacher, he now runs a well-known academy passing on his passion to future generations of barbers.

As a 14-year-old in New York, Sid Sottung worked in a barber's shop, learning the art of wet shaving and classic haircutting, trying it out on the shop's mostly Italian clientele. Soon, however, at his mother's behest, he moved into ladies' hairdressing, ending up working for Vidal Sassoon. He undertook their training program, learning how to create more contemporary looks for both men and women, but barbering was where his heart lay. Increasingly, he wanted to teach. At the age of 23, Sid moved out to Los Angeles and became a teacher for Vidal Sassoon, transferring to England to work in their advanced academy in London. A freelance career followed, styling hair for movie stars such as Tim Robbins and for catwalk models at events such as New York Fashion Week. But he still had the teaching bug and was making educational videos.

Life was not all rosy by this time, however, and after a period of decline, his life blighted by alcohol and drug abuse, he managed to change things around by doing what he loved most. "I was walking down a street one day," he explains, "and I saw this tiny shop. I thought it would be great for training, but even though I had only

about 43 cents in my pocket I signed the papers the next day. I had no idea how I was going to pay for it, but I called in a few favors, and by doing all the work myself I was able to launch a small training facility. Within eight months, I had to move to a bigger premises I was so busy. I changed my whole life around."

Indeed, he did. He now runs the Sid Sottung Academy in Nottingham, one of the country's premier educational facilities for barbers, teaching the craft of barbering to the next generation. He also teaches around the world, inspiring barbers wherever he wields his clippers.

He outlines his approach: "I like to take all different aspects of barbering techniques and mash it all together, taking ideas from the men's hairdressing side of things—working with men with long hair—using clippers, scissors, razors, and bringing in contemporary catwalk fashion. My ethos is to give the freedom to explore different ways of doing barbering, or wet shaving, or beard design. In the end, it's really what's going to work best for each individual student. Barbering is related to the fashion industry and fashion changes over time. So should hair and beard design."

New York to Nottingham
Sid Sottung, seen here in his trademark hat, is at the cutting edge of the industry. He's come a long way since learning from his mentor, a barber nicknamed "Bambino." His distinctive style inspires rookie barbers to present themselves with an air of panache.

ERIN WENTWORTH OF PALL MALL BARBERS
SHAVING AS MEDITATION

Erin is famed for offering one of the best shaves in London. Taught to shave the traditional way, she finds the whole process deeply calming, and when it's a Zen experience for the barber it follows that her clients must be the most blissfully relaxed gentlemen in town.

Fate can be a funny thing. That day, 13 years ago, if Erin Wentworth had not gone into work or had been on a different shift at the classy Mayfair barbershop, G. F. Trumper, where she worked reception, Britain might have been deprived of one of its finest barbers.

That morning, one of the younger barbers had turned up for work with a bit of stubble on his face after a heavy weekend. The manager of the establishment ordered him to shave at once, but the young barber, having taken a shine to his new look, refused. It was all half in jest, but the manager looked around his barbershop and told the young man that if he did not shave himself, he would get the receptionist, Erin, to shave him. Still the stubborn barber refused. So, the manager sat him down in a chair, and Erin was handed a cut-throat razor and a badger-hair shaving brush and told to shave him. She had no experience whatsoever

> "WE MAY BE A LITTLE MORE RELAXED IN OUR APPROACH TO GROOMING THESE DAYS. IT'S CERTAINLY CONSIDERED MORE OF A LUXURY TO GO TO A BARBER FOR A SHAVE—EITHER AS A RELAXING WAY TO FORGET ABOUT THE STRESSES OF LIFE OR AS PREPARATION FOR A SPECIAL EVENT, PERHAPS A MARRIAGE DAY."

with a razor, and it took her an hour, but she managed it without any cuts or nicks. Her boss, Mr. Stevens, who had supervised the shave, told her afterward: "You must capitalize on that; you'd be mad to sit on a reception desk."

Erin began to learn the art of barbering during her lunch hours, studied barbering at night-school and became a barber, all because of a bit of stubble and a stubborn young barber.

Erin Wentworth is now viewed as one of the country's top beard sculptors and traditional wet shavers, voted Best Shave in London by one magazine. She learned at Trumper's the old-fashioned way. "I was taught to do a traditional wet shave," she says. "That is, you shave from one side, you don't move from that spot. There's no running around the chair. You use one hand to shave. You use backhand on the other side of the face. It's a very old, traditional way to

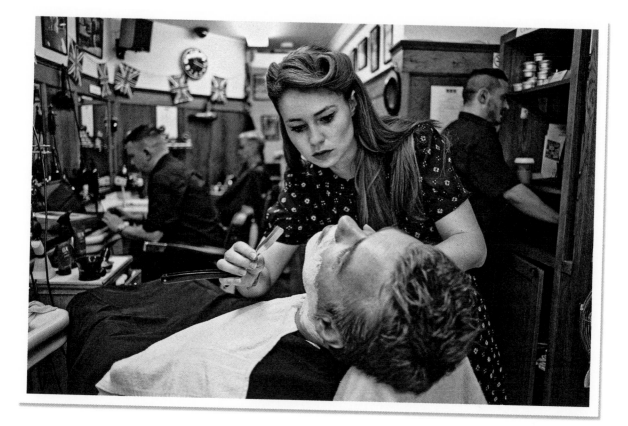

shave. You don't ask the client to do anything for you. You don't ask him to stick his chin out so you can get under his neck, you wouldn't ask him to stretch his top lip. Everything during that shave is done by you, while the client relaxes. You can lay somebody back in the chair, and he can relax, he can fall asleep, he can do as he wishes. I learned from a guy in his sixties who had been doing it that way for decades, and he had learned it from a guy who had been doing the same. But it still represents an important part of the male grooming tradition and makes a clear statement about the client's sense of self."

"I find it incredibly relaxing," she continues "I can be quite Zen. Which is why in a lot of photos of me while I'm shaving, I'm never looking at the camera. I'm always focused on what I'm doing. It's hard to explain. A lot of people find shaving very stressful because you've got a blade to somebody's face. For me it's like sometimes when you're walking down the road and when you arrive you forget how you got there. Sometimes it's so relaxing that at the end of a shave I don't remember doing it, although, of course, I'm very focused on the job in hand."

Shaving as meditation—now that's an interesting new concept.

Easy Does It
Erin, hailing from London's East End, seen here sporting a victory roll, is an aficionada of the "Peace in our time" vintage style for her own coiffeur. ✄

Erin Wentworth's Perfect Shave

Not so very long ago, a man might visit his barber once a week, as part of an important routine to look his neat and tidy best. As professionals, we must strive to give the best service when it comes to shaving, as it is traditionally the first and last word of being a barber.

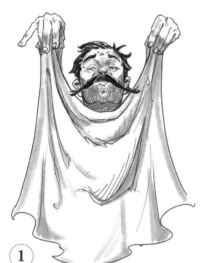

STEP ONE: To begin, we ensure our client is fully gowned up to prevent any spillage on his attire, and then he is reclined in the chair for the utmost comfort.

STEP TWO: I gently warm my hands in water and massage a pre-shave scrub into the bearded area. This will remove any impurities and ingrown hair. I leave the scrub on the face while I apply the first hot towel. This will open the pores and soften the facial hair. Then we use the hot towel to remove all the scrub from the face.

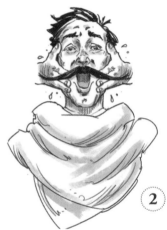

STEP THREE: Next, I use an oil to put a slight barrier between the skin and the blade to prevent any razor drag and condition the skin, gently massaging the oil into the skin, while paying special attention to any thicker/wiry parts of the beard. I apply a second hot towel to the face to enhance the effect of the oil and further soften the facial hair.

STEP FOUR: While the client has the second hot towel on, I whip up shaving cream into a luxurious creamy lather. I recommend using a badger hair shaving brush. Badger hair is extremely porous and holds heat better than a synthetic brush, which means more heat and water gets to the client's face. This will really lift the stubble off the face, leaving it standing up ready to be cleanly shaved away.

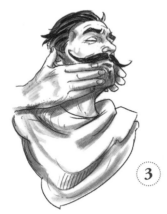

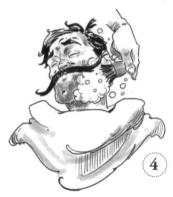

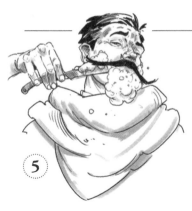

STEP FIVE: Using a freshly loaded open razor for shaving is a must. Let's face it, using a disposable safety razor in a luxury wet shave could be seen as cheating! Using confident strokes to remove the facial hair, I start to shave one side of the face from sideburn to jawline, always stretching the skin to prevent tugging on the face, slowly working around the chin and into the mustache area.

STEP SIX: As I was trained in the traditional art of shaving, I then use backhand razor strokes to shave the other side of the face, again shaving sideburn to jaw, until I come to the chin. Then finally the neck, using soft strokes, very gently, allowing my razor to do the work for me. I always leave the throat till last, for a personal flourish to finish. It is, after all, called a cut-throat shave! I strongly advise always shaving with the direction of the hair growth—this will lead to a more comfortable shave.

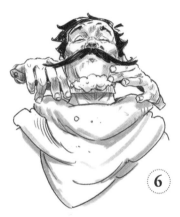

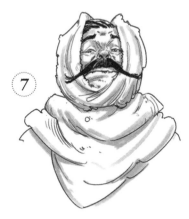

STEP SEVEN: To finish up a fantastically close shave, I recommend using another face wrap—this time with a cold towel—to close all the facial pores and to cool the face after it has been handled and shaved. The cold towel stage is especially helpful for those clients who have sensitive skin, as any redness or irritation experienced after such a close shave can be calmed and soothed as the client relaxes.

STEP EIGHT: To complete the shave, I always apply a moisturizer to the skin. One small tip when applying moisturizer is to not rub it into the skin as it can irritate the already stimulated face. Use your hands to gently pat the moisturizer onto the face. This will not only absorb and leave the skin hydrated, but smooth, soft, and silky to the touch.

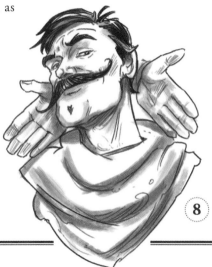

Barbering Treatments

From the Cosmic Barber of Pushkar, a slap-happy chappie of world repute, to the eye-watering molten beeswax used to remove nasal hair in Thailand, techniques vary from country to country. Thankfully bloodletting, leeches, and enemas are no longer on the menu. Rest assured, however, that time-honored barbering practises continue to offer a pleasurable experience, allowing gentlemen to face the world with renewed vigor.

THREADING

Threading is a hair-removal technique that originated in Asia and that has recently gained popularity in the West as a method for dealing with unruly facial hair. The practitioner takes a thin thread—probably of cotton or polyester—doubles it, knots the ends together, and twists it into an X shape, holding it at each end between spread fingers. It is then looped over the hair or line of hairs, and when one hand pulls the thread the hair is caught by the centre of the X of thread and pulled out. Some people use the mouth to hold the thread, and this method is said to be the fastest, most precise one. Threading is said to provide clearer definition where required and is gentler on the skin than other hair-removal methods. Done correctly, it need not be painful.

SINGEING

Singeing is an age-old technique, used for centuries to remove stray hairs. Turkish barbers are the masters of singeing, using it, for instance, to rid the ears of hair. Short, sharp tapping with a burning taper burns the hair without burning the client. It developed in response to the belief that hair contained fluid, and if it was singed to seal the hair ends that fluid was retained. Hair was viewed as a living part of the body and likely to bleed if it was cut. Singeing is said to bring a number of benefits—it seals split ends, closes the follicles, and is said to encourage hair growth. It also was claimed that sealing off the hair, thought to be hollow, prevented disease entering the body, just as cauterizing a wound stops bleeding.

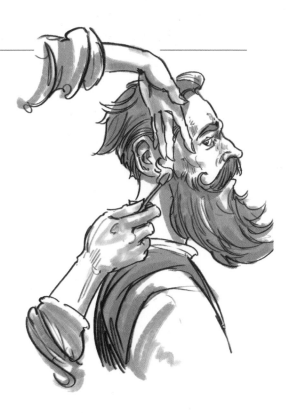

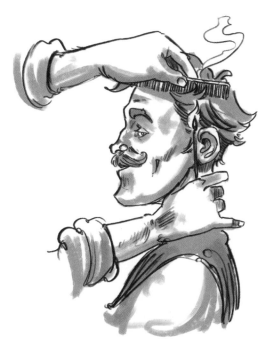

Traditionally, the singeing treatment involves running a candle or a dripless taper flame along twisted strands of hair to singe off stray and unhealthy ends. Flames are still commonly used today throughout the world in the process of ear hair removal. It was a technique commonly offered by itinerant barbers in the Middle East, as it involves simple, easily portable tools. Today, barbers who offer ear hair singeing point out the benefits of this ancient practice. They say that trimming unwanted ear hairs allow the ends to drop back into the ears, a source of itching and irritation and possible infection, whereas singeing leaves no debris behind, and is by its nature cleansing.

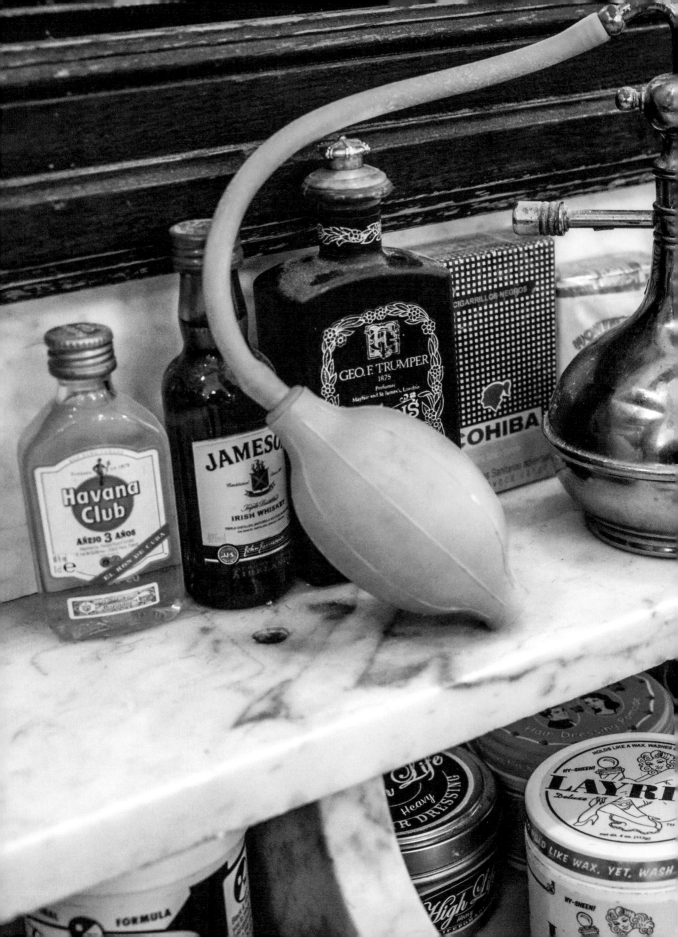

PERSONAL GROOMING

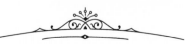

WITH THE FINEST TOOLS, UP-TO-DATE TECHNIQUES,
AND A WHOLE HOST OF DELECTABLE PRODUCTS, THE
MODERN GENTLEMAN TAKES TIME WITH HIS APPEARANCE.
PERSONAL GROOMING HAS NEVER BEEN SO LUXURIOUS.

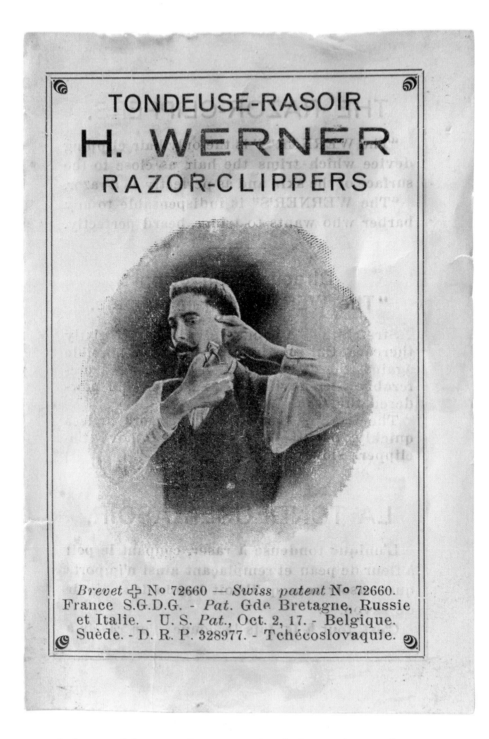

With the turn of the twentieth century and with the introduction of easier-to-use equipment, many men were encouraged to groom themselves.

MUCH AS I prize the egalitarian society of the barbershop, on occasion one desires solitude and serenity, an opportunity to reflect on the doings of the day and to prepare for the pleasures of the evening. While a shower and shave are undoubtedly a swift sharpener, be sure to allow some time to luxuriate in a foaming tub, recite some poetry, compose a speech, or rehearse a bawdy song ... out of mother's earshot.

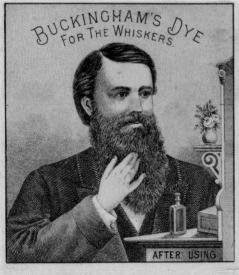

BUCKINGHAM'S DYE
FOR THE WHISKERS.

AFTER USING

*Those who desire to change the color of their beard and mustache to a beautiful **BROWN** or **BLACK** that will not wash off, will find our "**BUCKINGHAM'S DYE**" just the thing and very handy, being in one preparation.*

It is easy of application, safe and effectual, and is rapidly growing in public favor. Full directions on every bottle.

PREPARED BY

R. P. HALL & CO., Nashua, N. H.
Sold by all Druggists.   OVER

Powder and Paint

Along with the new-fangled razors and trimmers a whole host of products appeared on the market, all designed to enhance one's appearance (above and opposite). ❧

I N THE LAST 50 years or so, men have filled their bathroom cabinets with products to make them smell, look, and ultimately feel better. There are moisturizers, face scrubs, post-shave balms, anti-aging creams, and muscle-reviving body gels. Never has there been such a variety of lotions to soften the skin, manage the hair, preen the beard, and smooth wrinkles. There is fantastic equipment, too, with precision engineered safety razors, luxurious badger hair brushes, and combs designed specifically for the beard. Personal grooming no longer means a quick rub-down with a washcloth and a run of the fingers through the hair. The modern man takes time at his toilet.

Men have displayed their inner peacock for as long as they have been walking on two legs. We know that in 10,000 BC fragrant oils kept skin soft and body odors in check, and the Ancient Egyptians used gums, spices, and sweet-smelling plants. In the fourth century, Alexander the Great planted an Asian-inspired botanical garden in Athens to grow ingredients for exotic male beauty treatments, while acne-prone Romans dabbed barley flower and butter on annoying pimples and also, somewhat less charmingly, painted their nails with blood and sheep's fat.

Medieval physician Avicenna blended the arts of medicine and cosmetics in his writings, and apothecaries were consulted for dyes to cover gray hair and cures for baldness, such as onion juice and hog fat. Such vanities were frowned on by the powerful Church, which also spent a lot of time denouncing public bath-houses or "stewes," where bodies could have a good scrub but morals were harder to clean. Elizabethans were keen to disguise the ravages of time and scars of smallpox by applying egg and honey masks and bathing in red wine. The Victorians, while busy inventing things, cultivated beards, enabling them to pursue the Industrial Revolution without stopping to shave. Then in 1994, after attending an exhibition organised by *GQ* magazine, journalist Mark Simpson coined the phrase "Metrosexual Man." His prescience was unerring. "I'd seen the future of masculinity," he wrote, "and it was moisturized."

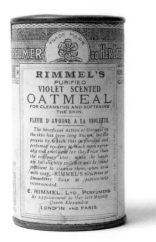

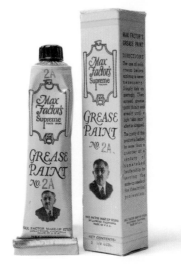

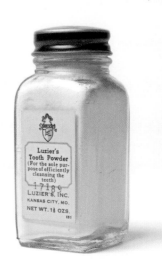

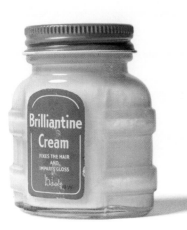

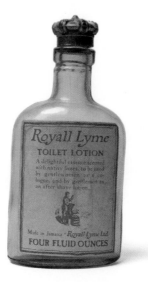

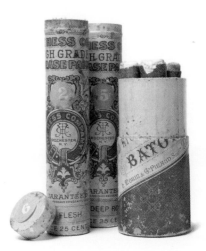

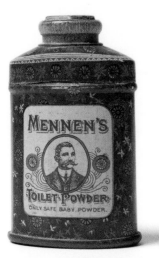

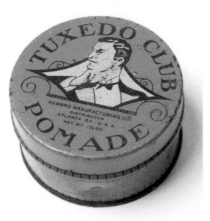

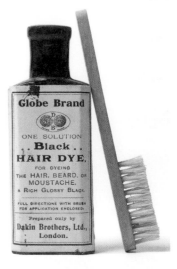

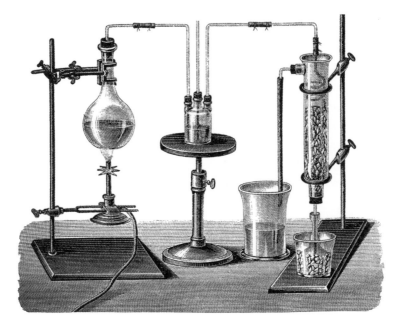

THE DARK ARTS

THE HEYDAY OF masculine make-up was surely the eighteenth century, although where beauty treatments were concerned it seems the Age of Enlightenment was anything but, and ingredients frequently had effects quite contrary to those promised. Recipe books explained how to make cosmetic preparations at home, and those commercially available were unregulated, untested, and often deadly.

The most significant fashion was for pale skin, and men pasted their faces with "ceruse" to whiten the complexion, cover smallpox scars, and conceal signs of ringworm. This toxic combination of lead and mercury blended with corrosive acids not only ravaged the skin but led to infertility, madness, and paralysis, long before the much sought deathly pallor became all too real.

The trend for excessive cosmetic adornment reached its pinnacle with the return of young fops fresh from their grand tour of Europe. Calling themselves Macaronis, they flaunted faces heavily painted in the French courtly style. However, the taste for such flamboyance was soon deemed unpatriotic, leading to the rejection of male make-up and no doubt contributing to a welcome improvement in gentlemen's health.

Animal, Vegetable, or Mineral?
Clockwise from top left: Portrait of a hog; antique leech jar; drawing of cochineal beetles crushed for carmine dye; advertisement for musky cologne; botanical sketch of belladonna or deadly nightshade squeezed into the eyes to dilate pupils; bottle of arsenic, which in wafer form was a popular Victorian cosmetic, despite being favored by contemporary murderers as their poison of choice. ❧

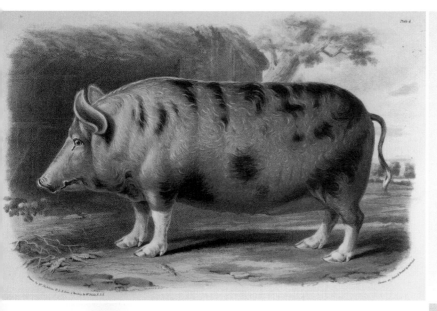

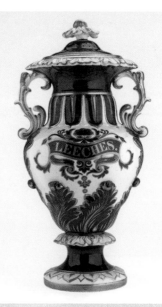

BEASTLY BEAUTY

——◆◆◆——

In days past, sourcing ingredients for cosmetics was the work of the alchemist and required no little ingenuity, perchance a degree of brutality. Potions including rendered pig fat, tinctures of deadly nightshade, mercury, the glandular secretions of deer, lead, and even crushed beetles would grace the dressing tables of the fashionista and the well-to-do.

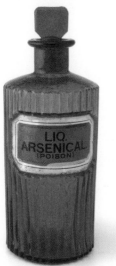

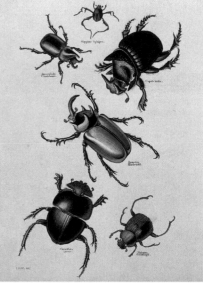

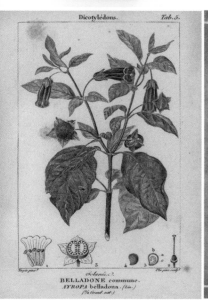

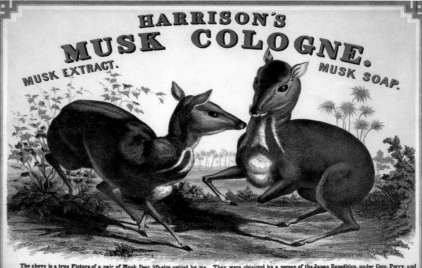

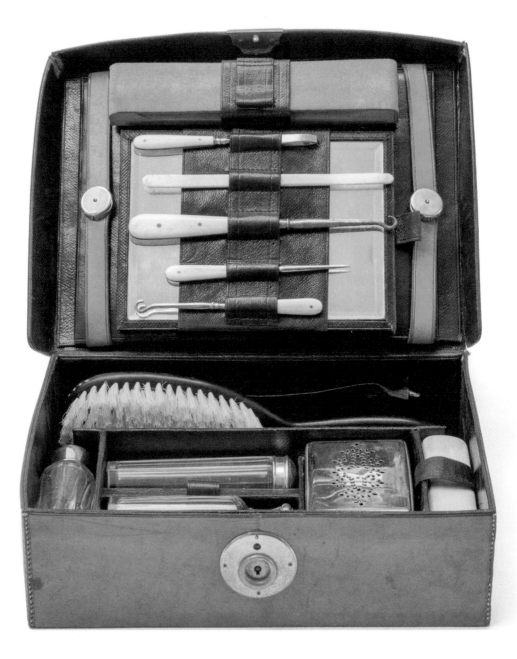

GENTLEMAN'S ESSENTIALS

The modern gentleman is likely to carry less than his historical counterpart,
who rarely traveled without a lavishly stocked dressing case. However, there are
some indispensable items one should never be without.

Traveling Kit

THE DRESSING CASE has its origins in the fourteenth-century French valise that contained the essentials for personal grooming and was used by traveling nobility and royalty. By the nineteenth century, the British were probably the world's greatest travelers, as exemplified by indomitable gentlemen such as Richard Burton and John Hanning Speke. Among the large amount of luggage and campaign furniture conveyed by bearers, railway porters, Sherpas, or a retinue of servants, the well-groomed explorer or soldier would carry a dressing case. This comprised a veritable treasure chest of what were deemed necessary grooming requisites, enabling him to look good, stay clean, and keep a stiff upper lip, regardless.

These cases contained an array of wonderful implements and tools, often monogrammed and made of ivory, ebony, mother-of-pearl, or tortoise-shell, with silver-topped cut-glass jars to transport colognes, pomades, and lotions.

These extravagant chests were made by eminent luxury goods manufacturers such as Drew & Sons, Jenner Knewstub, Mappin & Webb, Louis Vuitton, Cartier, Asprey, and Swaine Adeney. They were often constructed of exotic woods such as coromandel, rosewood, or walnut, and lined with satin, crushed velvet, or Moroccan leather.

Later, the introduction of plastics, coupled with the advent of air travel, resulted in smaller, more portable items often housed in leather cases, leading directly to the dopp kit or plastic bag containing the bare essentials we use today.

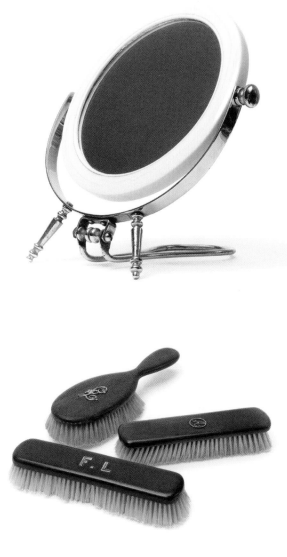

Reflecting Refinement
Exquisite, no-expense-spared items from the captain's personal collection. ❧

REQUISITES

A dressing case would typically contain:

hair brushes, clothes brushes, shaving brushes, razor, shaving soap, shaving strop, toothbrushes, tooth powder, glove stretchers, button hook, shoehorn, mustache curling tongs, spirit burner (for heating up the tongs).

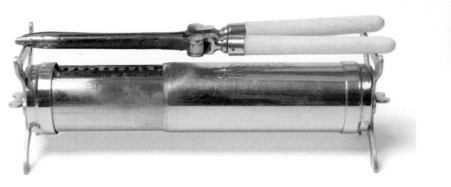

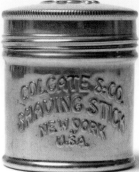

THE WHOLE KIT & CABOODLE

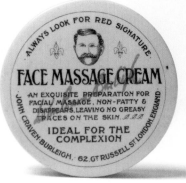

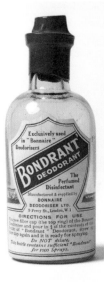

The Captain has found himself in many a sticky situation, but neither his resolve nor his mustache has ever drooped. To ensure he presents a brave face, he carries with him a selection of historic grooming items beautifully made from silver, pewter, ivory, ebony, leather, or fine porcelain.

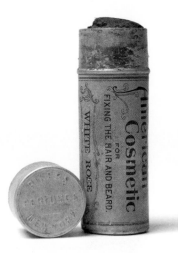

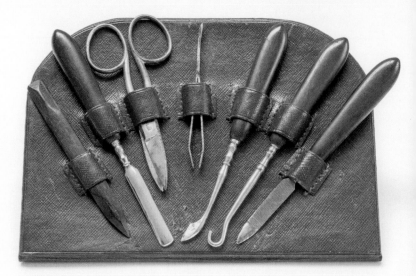

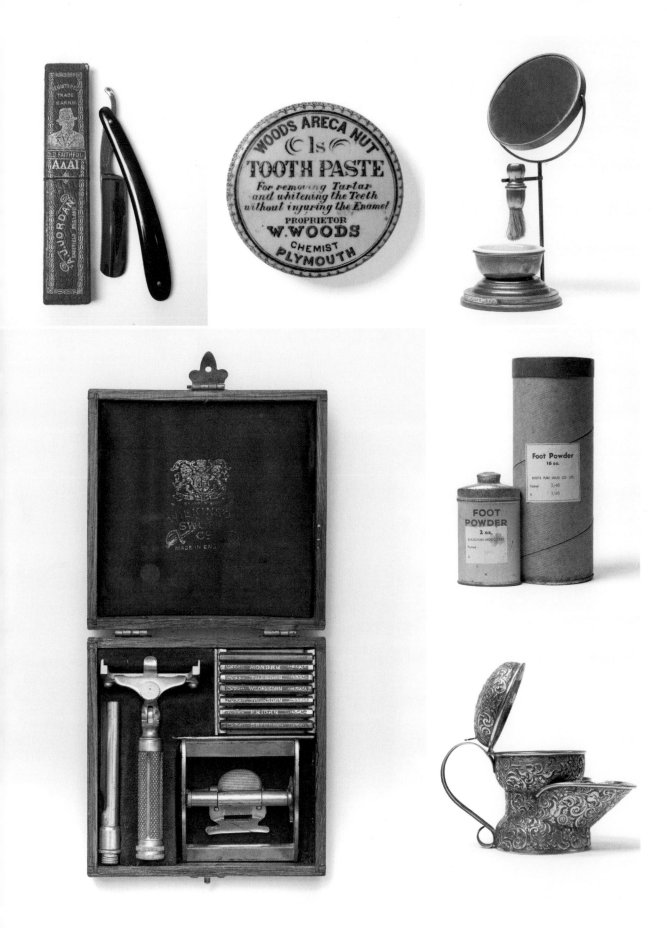

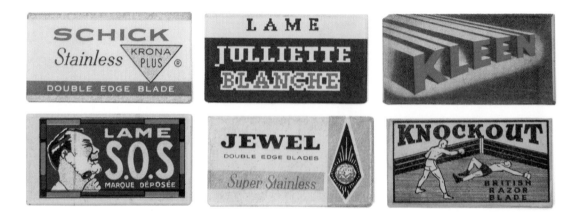

The Double-Edged Safety Razor

FRENCH MASTER CUTLER Jean-Jacques Perret is the author of the 1769 treatise *Pogonotomie, ou l'Art d'Apprendre à Se Raser Soi-Même* (*Pogonotomy, or the Art of Shaving Oneself*). Perret described a type of safety razor—a *rasoir à rabot,* or plane for the beard—that he had invented in 1762. Basing his idea on a carpenter's plane, he devised a razor with a wooden sleeve that enclosed the blade of a straight razor. Thus, only a tiny proportion of the blade showed, and the danger of the shaver wounding himself was greatly reduced.

Developments in shaving tools continued, and by the nineteenth century ideas more closely resembling our modern concept of the safety razor were emerging. In 1847, for instance, the English inventor William Samuel Henson came up with the first recorded version of the T-handled safety razor, with the blade perpendicular to the handle.

The extravagantly named American businessman King Camp Gillette, however, at the start of the twentieth century, made the double-edged safety razor an essential part of every man's grooming kit. Improving upon earlier designs, Gillette also introduced a cheaper razor steel blade, razor steel being a type of stainless steel designed specifically to be used in shaving. Patenting his tool in 1901, he began production in 1903, initially selling only a few

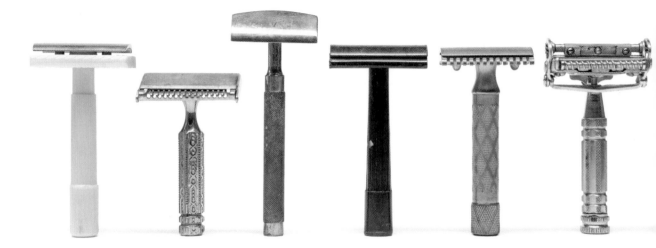

hundred blades and several dozen razors. In 1904, however, it took off; more than 90,000 razors and 123,000 blades were sold that year. By 1908, more than 1 million chins were being shaved using a Gillette razor. His products' growing domination of the market was confirmed by a contract with the U.S. armed forces during World War I. He supplied 3.5 million razors and a staggering 32 million blades.

The safety razor began to lose its pre-eminence with the introduction of better electric shavers and the proliferation of disposable branded razors such as Bic, Schick, Technomatic, Mach 3, and Fusion, among others.

Recently, however, renewed interest in male grooming has led to a fresh fascination with old-fashioned implements such as the cut-throat razor, and some manufacturers have even looked anew at the safety razor. Toronto-based Rockwell, for instance, raised the funding for their beautiful and revolutionary stainless steel razors via the crowd-funding website Kickstarter. The Rockwell Razor is a modern take on the double-edged safety razor, allowing the user to to select an angle of shaving most appropriate to his skin or hair growth.

More than 100 years on from the innovations of King Camp Gillette, the safety razor has well and truly entered a new era.

Sharp Design

Blades packaged in paper wraps (opposite above). A row of safety razors (opposite below). A gold-plated Gillette Aristocrat from 1930 (above). The innovative Rockwell Razor (below). ✴

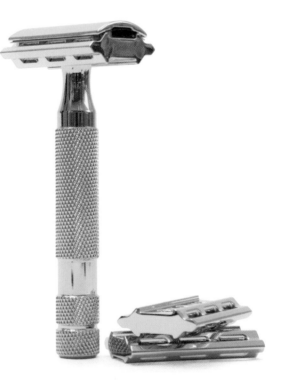

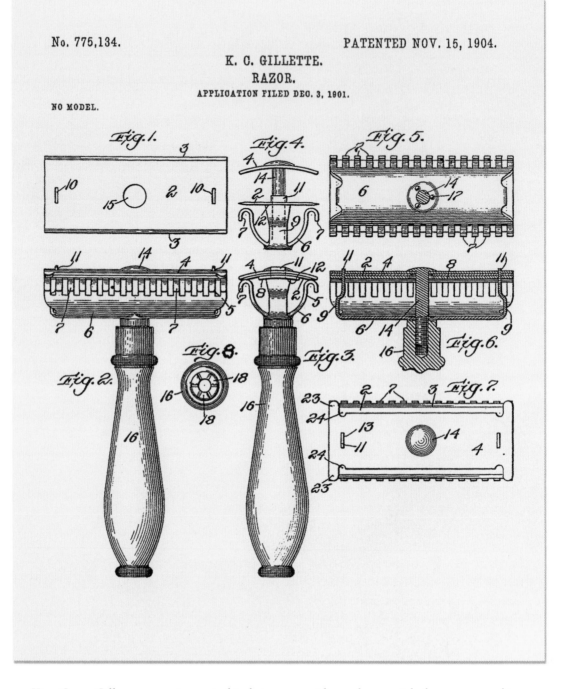

King Camp Gillette was a pioneer in his desire to provide gentlemen with the means to achieve a smooth safe shave in the comfort of their home. His invention unleashed a host of rivals.

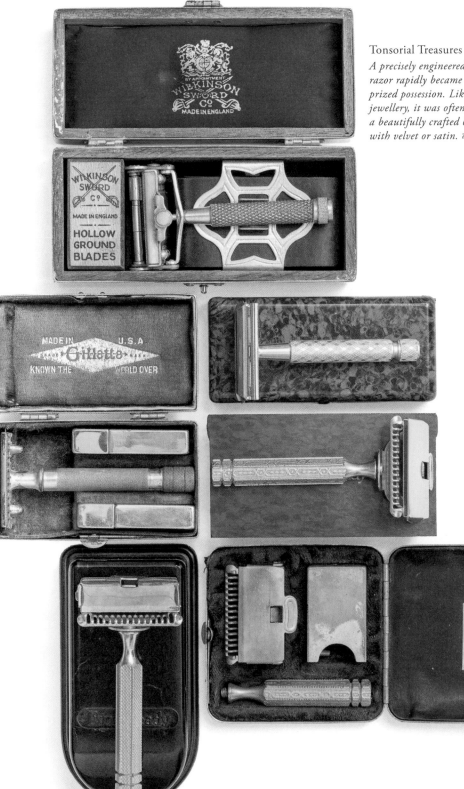

Tonsorial Treasures
A precisely engineered safety razor rapidly became a man's prized possession. Like a piece of jewellery, it was often housed in a beautifully crafted box lined with velvet or satin.

How to Shave with a Safety Razor

For most men shaving is a daily routine, and yet it's something that few have been taught, left instead to negotiate their early follicular flourishing alone by the bathroom mirror with nothing but an old razor found at the back of a cabinet. Smooth shaving is undoubtedly an acquired skill. Here is a recommended routine from the professionals:

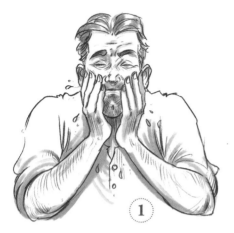

STEP ONE: *Wash*

The ideal preparation for a shave is a leisurely soak in a hot bath or a hot shower where one might also exercise the vocal chords. The steam will warm and clean the skin while softening the whiskers. A trained barber will use a hot towel to achieve the same effect. At home, if you have time, place a washcloth soaked in hot water over your face for a minute or two and indulge the quiet moment anticipating the joys of the occasion to come. If in an indecent hurry, at the very least wet your face with warm water to soften the whiskers.

STEP TWO: *Prepare the Skin*

This is vital and a step often missed when shaving at home. However, it will make an inestimable difference to the final smoothness of one's shave, so do not shirk! Which product to choose is a gentleman's preference, but in the captain's experience the best results are achieved using shaving oil. A small amount poured into the palm of one hand and then massaged gently into clean, warmed cheeks and chin creates the perfect base for the next step.

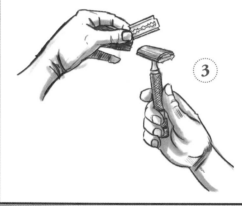

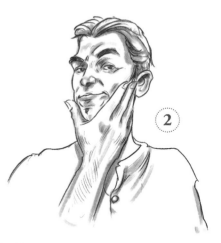

STEP THREE: *Prepare the Razor*

It's as possible to achieve a "baby's bottom" smooth shave with a double-edge safety razor as with a skilled barber's cut-throat. The blades of the razor must be bathed in hot water before shaving and the lather frequently washed off either under a tap or in a basin to keep the blades clean. Disassemble your safety razor and insert the blade. If you're using an adjustable razor, then set your razor to your preferred setting.

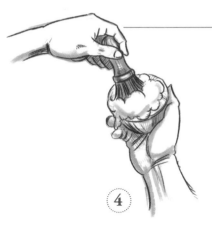

STEP FOUR: *Lather*

Now, as the ads claim, it's quick enough to squirt on foam from an aerosol can. But a small amount of good-quality shaving cream or soap mixed in a bowl each day is economical, and, for gents keen on doing their bit for the environment, this is infinitely preferable to discarding several cans of aerosol shaving foam to achieve a lesser result. A good-quality badger hair brush has the added advantage, if wielded with appropriate vigor, of lifting the hairs and stimulating the skin.

STEP FIVE: *The Shave*

Place your loaded safety razor against your skin at a 45-degree angle. There's no need to apply pressure to the razor or press it into your skin—simply let the weight of the razor do the work for you as it glides across your skin, shearing off your facial hair. For best results, shave with the grain or your stubble. A professional barber might go over a chap's chin a second time and will shave each area twice, once in each direction. As a gentleman becomes acquainted with his own visage, he will discover which direction gives the best results, and it may well vary as he traverses the valleys and contours of his own profile. In most cases, it is unnecessary to go over the whole face a second time, although in pursuit of a perfect finish certain areas might stand to benefit from double the attention.

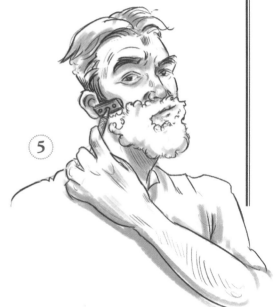

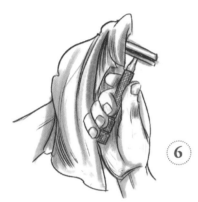

STEP SIX: *Clean*

When certain a good clean shave has been achieved, it's essential to wash one's face thoroughly in clean water. Patting the face with cool or cold water is an excellent way to calm the skin and close pores opened by the hot water. Fellows susceptible to spots and the odd slip of a blade may need to invest in a styptic pencil or an alum block, which will help close up small cuts. Apply a moisturizing post-shave balm. Finally, be sure to dry your razor with a cotton or micro-fiber towel, and store it in a secure place to ensure the longevity of your essential shaving tool.

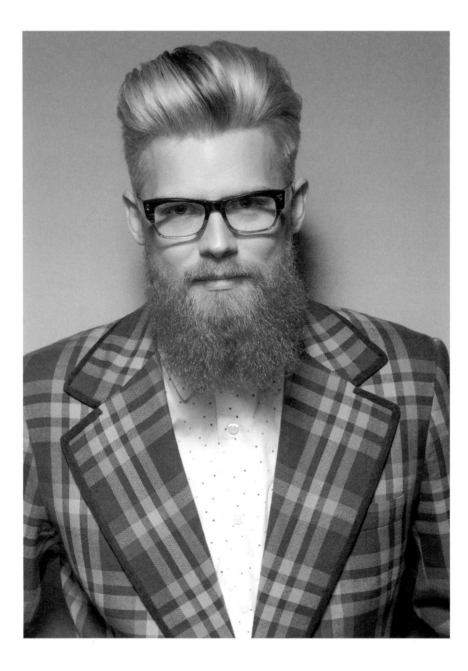

SPRUCING UP

A well-turned-out chap looks healthy, and clear skin and well-tended hair not only look smart but lift one's mood and enhance self-esteem. Making oneself presentable is good form socially and is vital to the self-respect of a confident gentleman.

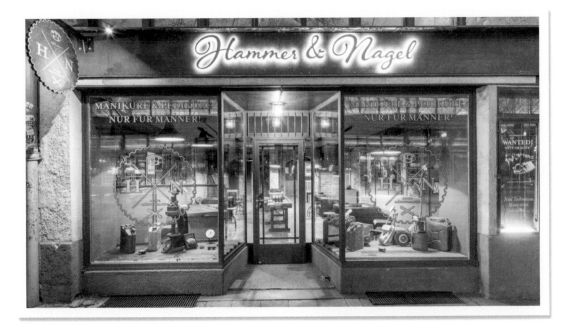

Making an Impression

THE MODERN GENTLEMAN has embraced grooming with, some might observe, an ardor surpassing that of his historical counterparts.

In the interests of enterprise, a recent study of gentlemen and their grooming products found that in America and the U.K., fellows are devoting a substantial part of their hard earned income to sprucing themselves up. We lag slightly behind the ladies (as is only polite) who are more extravagant by between 35 to 40 percent, but feminine statistics include cosmetics alongside general skincare products, inflating the bill by a pretty penny.

The twenty-first-century gentleman might also be found perusing the dressing table of his wife or girlfriend and borrowing an item or two. The trend for keeping up appearances is also evident from the proliferation of new barbershops across the world. There is no doubt, men are devoted to grooming.

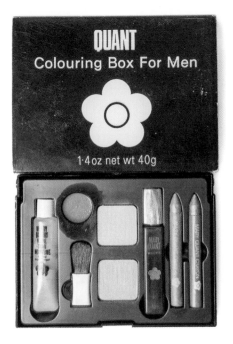

Men Only
A modern gentlemen's nail bar (top). Make-up for men?
Mary Quant was always ahead of the curve (above).

Your Personal Regime

A fellow eager to transform from charming scruff to dapper Dan often asks, "How on Earth can I hone my appearance?" How indeed! It takes commitment, practice, and consistency of effort. A would-be gentleman needs to experiment and discover what works for his own features.

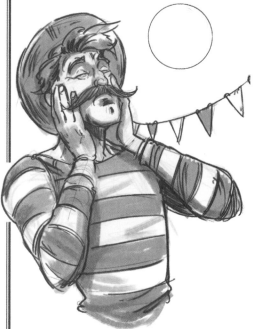

SKINCARE

After shaving, it is extremely important to moisturize the skin. Find a product that doesn't irritate when your face is freshly shaved and "raw." The ideal moisturizer should have some protection from the sun included (code name: SPF). This is of utmost importance all year round as the sun's harmful effects are not limited to the halcyon days of high summer. The modern gentleman can confidently admit to taking care of his complexion. If unsure of your skin type, consult a professional, although different levels of dryness or greasiness are usually obvious, as is the impact of one's living and working conditions or changing seasons and climates. Attention paid to the skin, keeping it clean, moisturized, and protected all year round, will reward the modern gentleman with a healthy glow and youthful looks long into maturity.

HAIR

His hair is one of the most visible aspects of a gentleman's approach to grooming. Ensuring it is well cut, styled, and clean at all times will mark you as a modish man about town or a polished country gent. We explore the fascinating science behind our follicular forestation in the next chapter. Suffice it to say here that one must establish a regular relationship with one's barber. It is possible to spend a great deal on a haircut, but what matters most is finding a barber who is liked and trusted and who cuts hair as a gentleman requests and within his budget. Set a grooming schedule and stick to it. This is likely to be every four to six weeks, unless one is a thespian preparing for the role of Tarzan, Edgar Rice Burroughs's feral hero.

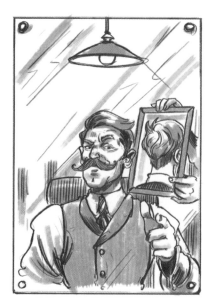

TEETH

It must be observed that a chap requiring a reminder to brush his teeth has a long road to travel before claiming to be a gentleman. Poor oral health may prove ruinous in business and romance. Regular visits to a dentist and hygienist ought to have been part of one's routine since childhood, so if this has been allowed to slide, book an appointment, turn up, and follow the advice of the experts. Modern dentistry can do much to improve a snaggletoothed smile and repair the knocks of sporting mishaps or bouts of fisticuffs, so rest assured that your dentist will have seen worse.

MANICURES & PEDICURES

The assumption that pampering the hands and feet remains the preserve of women proves to be the Achilles heel of many an aspiring gentleman. After all, the care of the feet is part of any athlete's routine and not to be sniffed at. Even if one's sporting prowess is proudly amateur, unless one's hands are permanently enveloped in gloves the digits will not escape attention, and a gentleman must ensure his nails are well maintained and ready for a firm friendly handshake at any time. Of course, the process of soaking, filing, tidying the cuticles (taking care not to cut living skin), buffing, and moisturizing can be undertaken at home. Most men omit polish, but each to his own—after all, throughout history men have colored their nails. However, the benefits of a professional consultation are manifold. A trained technician will give guidance on infections and problems like ingrown toenails, the removal of corns, and trimming of nails as well as advice on overcoming bad habits such as nibbling and picking at cuticles. The hands and feet give good service and are used all the time, so it's good to make sure they look and feel their best.

TO CONCLUDE: *A gentleman must plan and refine to succeed. Following a simple daily routine, whether at home, overnighting at the mother-in-law's, or zigzagging up the Zambezi in a dug-out canoe, will ensure one begins the day bright-eyed, bushy-tailed, and with a certain spring to the step.*

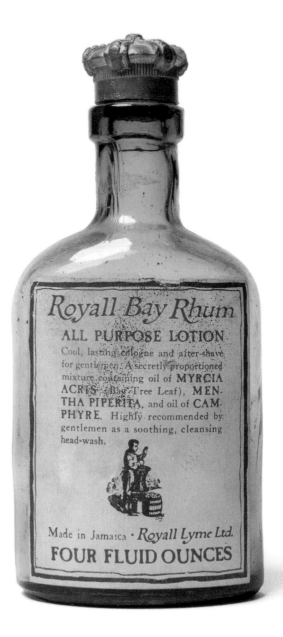

CROWNING GLORY

The way you wear your hair makes an immediate and powerful statement about you and how your perceive yourself. The hair cuticle is also an accurate barometer of your health, habits, and recent history. Time to brush up on your behavior.

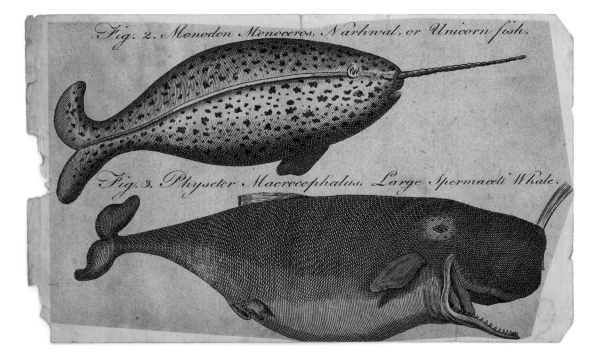

Shampoo

HAIR IS DEAD; long live hair. The action all takes place under your skin at the base of the hair follicle, and once it is grown out it cannot really get any better. This is where shampoo comes in, designed to give dull or dirty hair a bit of a bounce or a charming gleam.

We have India to thank for shampoo, and the very word is derived from the Hindi word *chāmpo*. As early as the sixteenth century, the Indians were mixing the pulp of the soapberry with a few herbs and flowers to keep their hair looking good, and British traders to the subcontinent returned with the fresh new idea of shampooing the hair. In those days, hair was rarely washed more than once a month, if at all, and it was only in the early twentieth century that regular hair-washing became common. In the late 1920s, liquid shampoo came along, and a hair-wash became less of a chore.

As a detergent, commercial shampoos are not particularly good because they strip the hair of its natural oils. Conditioner, therefore, is recommended for reducing such damage.

Dry shampoo has come very much into vogue of late, reviving a product that dates back to the late fifteenth century when Asian peoples cleaned their hair with clay powder. It has become popular once again because not only does it save time but it also saves water, making it good for the environment, and it protects hair against loss of color and nutrients.

A Whale of a Time
An engraving of a sperm whale. An organ in the mammal's head contains some 440 gallons of a pearly white waxy substance called spermaceti, from which a sweet-smelling oil is produced that was once used in cosmetics and pharmaceuticals. ❧

Hair Today, Gone Tomorrow

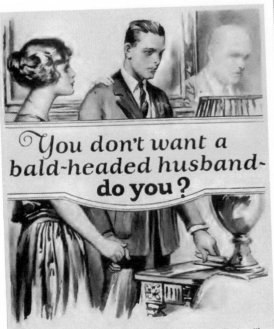

You don't want a bald-headed husband—do you?

YOUR husband will be either bald or good-looking. It's largely up to you.

You know more than he does about the care of hair. Most of the fairer sex know that a healthy scalp *keeps* its hair. Millions of women know that Wildroot Hair Tonic does more than lend a lustrous lure to the hair—it keeps the scalp healthy.

But your husband (or husband-to-be)—he may think that *after* he gets bald, he can then use some hair-restorer and get his looks back again. But *you* know that there is nothing that will cure baldness—just as you know that the proper care of hair

with Wildroot Hair Tonic will help *prevent* baldness.

It seems strange that intelligent men do not realize these simple facts. A woman realizes them because she studies them. And she knows that much of her charm either as a wife or as a wife-to-be depends upon the attractiveness of her coiffure.

You probably have Wildroot Hair Tonic in your own boudoir. If you haven't it, your druggist will gladly supply you. You will want to use it regularly to keep *your* hair lovely, and you will want your husband to use it to help him *avoid* bald-headedness. Wildroot Co., Inc., Buffalo, N. Y.

WILDROOT HAIR TONIC

The Bald Truth
As this 1924 advertisement for Wildroot Hair Tonic shows, hanging on to one's hair was deemed socially and romantically advantageous, so men looked to obscure cures for hair loss—or their wives did. ❧

OF COURSE, WHATEVER unguents we choose to apply to our hair, health, exercise, and nutrition play a major part in healthy hair growth, whether on the head or of the facial variety. What you consume not only affects your hair's health, but is recorded in the strands themselves, as respected trichologist, Professor Barry Stevens, explains: "Hair is a book, it's history. Certain things you eat will be documented for as long as the hair remains. It will be chronicled that you took that drug or drank that drink or ate that food and the record is accessible as long as that section of hair exists." Abstain from narcotics, drink, and ordering in pizza, therefore. Your diet should be healthy and nutritious and must be rich in vitamins and proteins if you want a healthy scalp and facial hair. There are, of course, supplements that claim to encourage facial hair growth, but the captain would advise you to give those a wide berth and watch out for what Professor Stevens describes as "charlatans, fraudsters, posturers, and snake-oil salesmen."

Another piece of bad news is that, like the doornail debated by Charles Dickens in *A Christmas Carol*, hair is most emphatically dead. As soon as it pushes out through your skin it is no longer a living thing. As Professor Stevens told us: "There is no blood supply to it; therefore, it is dead." It also lacks nerves and muscles, and, of course, when it is cut, its owner feels no pain. It is still rather amazing, however. Made of keratin, a fibrous protein, it is built from cells like those of our skin. Each hair grows from a single follicle and at the base of the follicle is the Papilla. This is the bud of the hair and it is there that the majority of the hair's growth takes place. Each shaft of hair is made up of three layers: the outer Cuticle, made up of overlapping layers: the Cortex, which contains the hair's main bulk and its color; and the Medulla, which is a thin core made up of transparent cells and air spaces.

Of course, many men long for those follicles to be working properly and there is evidence that baldness has been a cause of anxiety for the well-groomed male throughout history. Four millennia ago, the Egyptians were searching for a cure for baldness, and they employed some fairly disgusting ingredients in their cures, including the fats of various unfortunate animals, alabaster, the toes of a dog, and the hoof of an ass. Hippocrates, the Greek "father of modern medicine," was bald and invented several treatments including one containing a mixture of horseradish, cumin, pigeon droppings, and nettles that was applied vigorously to the scalp.

Our resident trichologist, Professor Stevens insists that if you suffer the typical hair loss of men around the age of 40 to 50, there is not a lot that can be done, unless you go for the hair transplant option. "Around the age of 45 to 50, you get a slow change in the structure of the follicle brought about by the presence of an androgen, a male hormone, usually testosterone. That causes the miniaturization of scalp hair

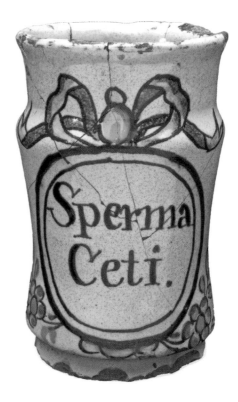

Prized for Pomade

Being extremely difficult to obtain, spermaceti (literally "whale seed") oil, was expensive, highly prized, and carefully stored in decorative pots such as this earthenware jar, thought to be from early nineteenth-century Italy (above). Modern preference for grooming ingredients leans more to plant-based extracts, such as jojoba oil. ❧

BEARD TALK

Pogon is Greek for beard and is the root, if you will excuse the pun, of these important words referring to facial hair:

Pogonophile: an aficionado of the beard, or a reader of *The Gentleman's Guide to Grooming*

Pogonophilia: the love and admiration of the beard

Pogonophobia: a fear of beards

Pogonotomy: shaving

Pogonotrophist: a barber, or a person who grooms, sculpts, or trims beards

Pogonotrophy: the art of growing and cultivating a beard

follicles in certain areas. Strangely enough it falls within the hat line in the male and, oddly, all over the scalp in the female. That is where all the rot comes in, the miracle cures. They're not miracle cures at all, in fact there aren't any cures."

However there are measures we can take to keep our locks lustrous while we have them. For gentlemen who shower regularly (and unless one is halfway up the Ubangi or deep undercover, there is no excuse to avoid regular ablutions), a regular hair wash is highly likely. Be warned! This frequency may be excessive, particularly with a strong shampoo. Try washing hair less often to retain natural oils and increase its health and vitality. Regular conditioning after washing will greatly improve the quality and manageability of even the most rebellious thatch. Hair today, gone tomorrow, as they say, and that is the way it will probably remain.

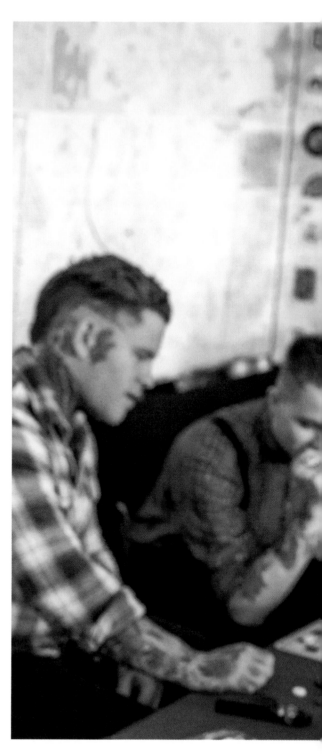

Chairmen of the Board
Strategic skills derived from a game of poker, draughts, dominos, or chess have been valued by soldiers, boxers, mathematicians, and magicians since antiquity. Here, modern gentlemen are partaking in convivial mental sharpening while waiting for the barber. ❧

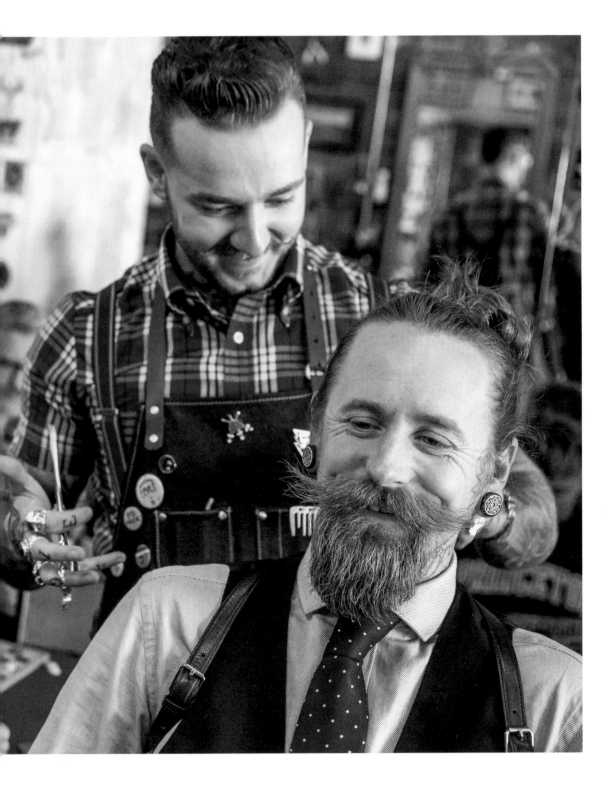

How to Grow a Beard

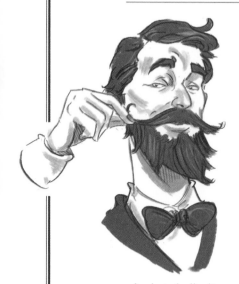

It's the perennial question. "How can I make my beard grow faster, thicker, longer?" We're very sorry to have to tell you that you can't. You see, all human hair grows at the same rate, about $\frac{1}{2}$ inch a month. Despite a plethora of products that claim otherwise, you cannot make it grow faster. Our good friend Professor Stevens warns that only age may provide a bit of a spur: "All you can do is get older, because around a man's fortieth year your beard hair will grow at a faster rate than ever before." There is, however, something called terminal beard length. There are different types of hair—vellus/languo hair is the downy kind that covers most of our bodies. Primary terminal hair is our eyebrows and eyelashes. Secondary terminal hair, however, is everything else—chest, legs, arms, scalp, face, and down below. The keratinized cells in the hair follicle keep it growing. Beards average about two years, but when it stops for a rest the follicle shrinks and the hair bulb disappears. About 1 percent of your hair is doing this at any one time. Then there is the telogen phase, during which the hair falls out. As Beardsgaard Barbers say: "Just remember that growing your beard is a journey, not a destination. It will go through phases where it doesn't seem to be making much progress, then growth picks up again."

LET IT GROW, LET IT GROW, LET IT GROW Do not shave for at least six weeks. This will reveal where your beard growth is strongest. It is best to avoid any trimming or shaping at this stage, however tempting, so leave well alone.

EAT A WELL-BALANCED DIET As we have discovered from the experts, your hair is an accurate statement of both your lifestyle choices and state of health, so treat it well.

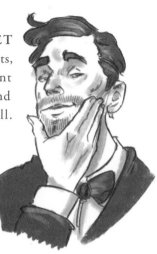

SOOTH INEVITABLE IRRITATION If within this initial period of experimentation your face becomes a tad itchy, moisturize your stubble with a good quality beard oil. But rest assured you will grow through this irritation.

DON'T FALL AT THE FIRST As such, ignore any disparaging remarks made by your mother, friends, partners, or colleagues! Carry on!

GENTLY BRUSH YOUR BEARD Applying a real wild boar bristle brush to the emerging beard on a daily basis will stimulate the growth.

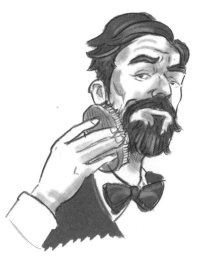

VISIT A REPUTABLE BARBER An adept facial hair stylist will be able to sculpt your beard to suit your face shape, the cut of your jib, and your individual beard hair growth pattern.

AVOID SHAMPOOING YOUR BEARD This can strip the hair cuticle of its natural oils. I would also advise against use of a hairdryer as this is likely to dry out the hair further, causing it to become brittle and the hairs to possibly break.

APPLY BEARD OIL TO WET HAIR Then comb through to enrich and condition while adding a beautiful sheen to your pride and joy.

USE A LIGHT MOUSTACHE WAX This can train the hair up and away from your upper lip.

COAX, CAJOLE AND REWARD In truth, combining patience and careful nurturing, along with gentle persuasion, cannot help but achieve great results.

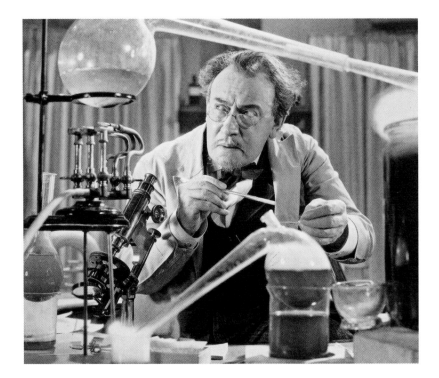

CREATE YOUR OWN

HAIR TREATMENTS

THE MODERN GENTLEMAN is a knowledgeable fellow, well informed about the provenance of the food he eats and the products he uses. He can whip up an omelette or mix an elegant cocktail, and now he can turn a nonchalant hand to crafting his own hair treatments.

In the days before cosmetics were mass-produced, a gentleman made the best of himself with whatever ingredients were at hand. The recipes opposite reflect traditional preparations adapted with a twist of contemporary spice, much like the captain's own. They can be made with natural ingredients easily sourced by the modern gentleman from the kitchen or bathroom cabinets or online for the more specialized stuff. One need not be a man of science to follow the simple recipes, although if a lab coat and goggles have sartorial appeal, feel free to indulge. Likewise, bunsen burners may be reserved for the lighting of cigars.

There is nothing worse than the wilting of one's carefully crafted pompadour or quiff, so may we present two lightly fragranced pomades along with a delectable bay rum hair tonic. We should indicate these recipes are for personal use or passing on to favored friends but not to be sold, no matter how the general public might try to persuade a fellow to divulge his secrets.

BAY RUM

Bay rum is a fresh hair tonic with a scent recalling the warm, spiced air of the West Indies. One would advise against consumption, although the captain highly recommends reserving a tot of said rum for imbibing, should a sea voyage be on the horizon.

INGREDIENTS

Dark Jamaica rum 10%
Formulator's alcohol 50%
Demineralized water 37.5%
Bay oil 2%
Pimento leaf oil 0.5%

REQUIRED EQUIPMENT

Measuring scale ❧ Heatproof glass jug ❧ Metal spoon ❧ Plastic pipette *(optional)* ❧ Plastic wrap ❧ Bottle with cap

METHOD

Place the glass jug on the measuring scale before setting the counter to zero. Add the ingredients in the order above. If you have essential oils in bottles with dropper inserts, you can measure the essential oils by drops. If not, you can use a disposable plastic pipette for each oil.

Stir the mixture well to ensure the ingredients fully combine. The liquid will be opaque and have a brown tint from the rum. You may notice a slight heady odor of alcohol when the product is freshly made. Fear not, for all is well. Cover the jug with the plastic wrap and leave in a safe place to macerate for around 5 days, at which point the bay rum is ready to use. Transfer to a clean, sterilized bottle and seal.

POMADE

Pomade was originally produced from animal fat and was prone to becoming rancid. In a bid to mask the increasingly unpleasant odor, early recipes were often scented with pulped fruit, which, from the French word *"pomme"* for apple, led directly to the hair product's name.

INGREDIENTS

Unrefined coconut oil 20%
Castor oil 59%
Beeswax 20%
Lime oil 1%

REQUIRED EQUIPMENT

Measuring scale ❧ Heatproof glass jug ❧ Metal pan ❧ Thermometer ❧ Metal spoon ❧ Plastic pipette *(optional)* ❧ Glass jars with lids

METHOD

Place the glass jug on the measuring scale and weigh the ingredients in the order given above, except for the essential oil.

Place the heatproof jug in a pan of simmering water and heat to 140 to 160°F, allowing the ingredients to melt completely before removing the pan from the heat.

Wait for the mixture to cool to around 100 to 115°F, when it will start to become slightly hazy. Add the essential oil, either from a bottle with a dropper or using a pipette. Stir to combine, pour into clean, sterilized jars, and seal.

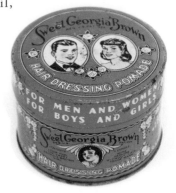

A Vintage Pomade
First made in the 1940s, Sweet Georgia Brown has been sold ever since. Packaged in distinctive red tins barely changed from the original design, it is still popular today.

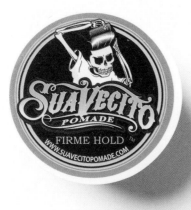
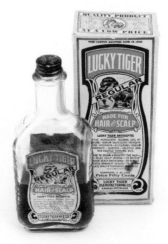
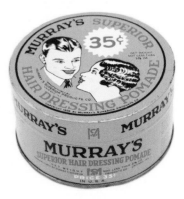
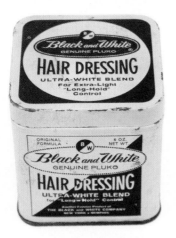
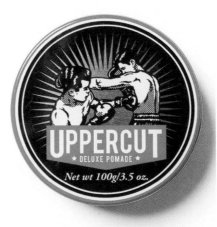
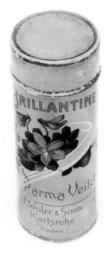
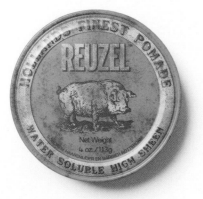
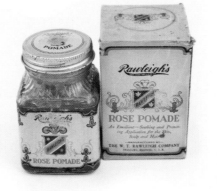
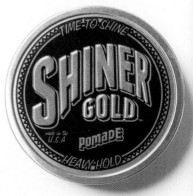

Original Teenage Rebels

"Teddy Boys" interpreted Edwardian fashions re-introduced by post–World War II Savile Row tailors. Flaunting pomaded pompadours, they carried steel combs to maintain slick quiffs and taper their hair to the shape of a duck's tail feathers. Only squares thought DA stood for district attorney.

PETER SWORDS KING
MOVIE INDUSTRY BIG-WIG

For more than 35 years, Oscar-winning hair and make-up designer Peter Swords King has enjoyed an extraordinary career bringing movie characters to life by ensuring they look right for the period and the character when they are in front of the camera.

A former wig-maker, Peter found his way into film via the theater, working first at the Bristol Old Vic before forming a wig-making company and then landing the position of wig and hair stylist on Peter Greenaway's sumptuous late seventeenth-century murder mystery, *The Draughtsman's Contract*. "It had big wigs in it!" he laughs. "Another film followed and another and another, and that's what I've been doing now for God knows how many years." He has worked on around 40 films, and among his credits are Jane Campion's *Portrait of a Lady*, starring Nicole Kidman and John Malkovich, *Velvet Goldmine*, with Ewan McGregor and Christian Bale, a couple of *Pirates of the Caribbean* films, the three *Lord of the Rings* films, and *The Hobbit* trilogy. He won an Oscar in 2003 for his work on *The Lord of the Rings: The Return of the King*. He has done period work, a film set in the glam rock period, and has even managed to turn six people, including Heath Ledger, Richard Gere, and Cate Blanchett, into Bob Dylan in *I'm Not There*.

> "MY JOB IS BASICALLY TO HELP PEOPLE BELIEVE THE STORY. YOU REALLY SHOULDN'T NOTICE THE HAIR OR THE MAKE-UP. YOU SHOULD JUST BELIEVE THE CHARACTER."

The hair and make-up designer's work is critical in the direction a film can take, and actors often look to the work of an expert like Peter to guide them in their characterization. There are also continuity issues because films are rarely shot in chronological order. The use of wigs and fake beards makes life a lot simpler, however. "We use human hair for wigs but sometimes with beards it's yak hair. The yak's belly hair is softer, and top yak is quite coarse. If I want a fine beard I use human hair, and it's always human hair on the edges because you get a nice fine line."

Nowadays, with high definition and 4K resolution, precision is the name of the game. As Peter explains, shooting in these formats provides a kind of hyper-reality, to the extent that a filter has to be added afterwards to make it look like film! "We have to be precise down to the individual hair. Especially on *The Hobbit*, which was shot at 48 frames per second, giving very high definition. One hair out of place and it's immense on screen."

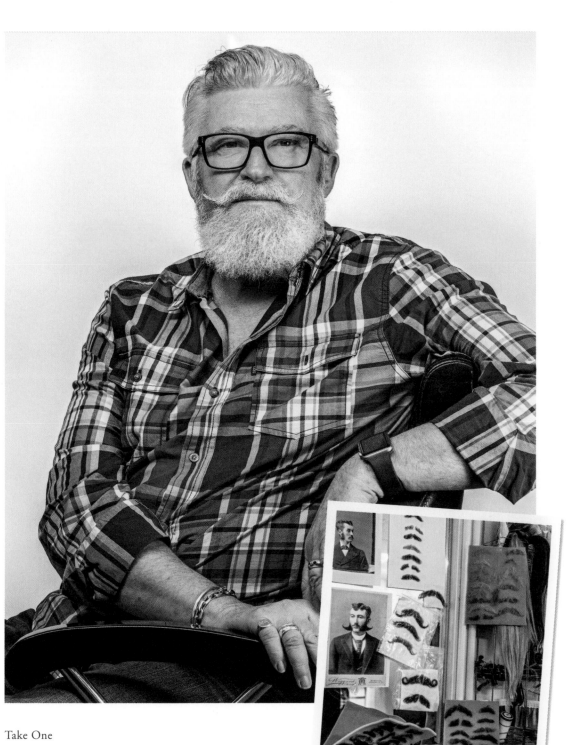

Take One

Peter Swords King, who as the creative director of the Bath Academy of Media Makeup instructs students in the skillful application of facial hair, ensures that actors will be able to maintain a stiff upper lip, regardless. ✺

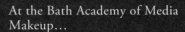

At the Bath Academy of Media Makeup…

…Tom Russell volunteered to allow Peter Swords King to demonstrate his barbering expertise by sacrificing his beloved beard while fundraising for the Young Minds' Trust. The captain is delighted to report that Tom's facial follicles are now flourishing once again after his brief foray into the short back and sides.

TRANSFORMATION

Here we see Peter Swords King taking Tom through a sequence of historical styles. What a difference the hair makes!

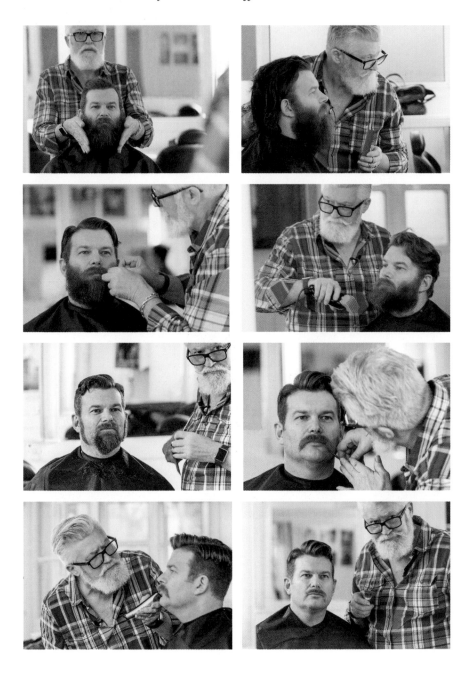

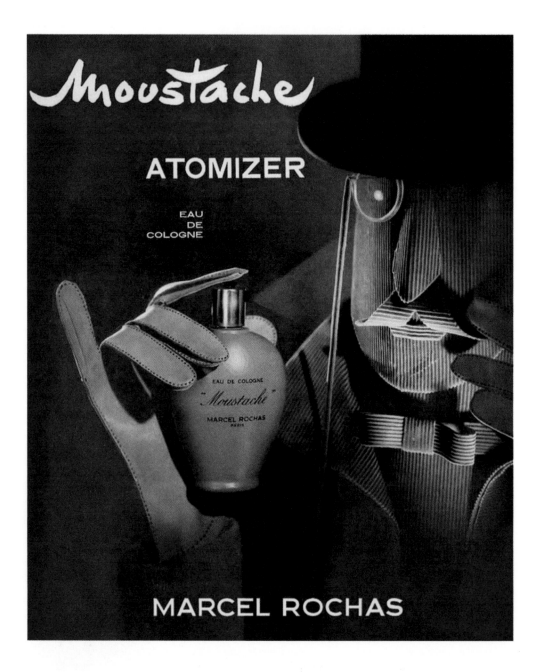

PERFUME

A gentleman's fragrance is exceptionally important. The days of the overpowering aftershave are gone. Advertisers would have you believe you need a powerful body spray to guarantee romantic success. In truth, it is better to use fragrance sparingly and subtly.

Perfume's Beginnings

PERFUME IS INTENSELY potent, evoking moments and memories with a piercing precision beyond the power of words. It's practical too—after all, humans have been intent on disguising the natural odors of the body for millennia.

Our knowledge of perfume's history begins about 6,000 years ago. We know that perfume was used in China, and the use of scent came to Europe via India, but the first written information is provided by the Ancient Egyptians, who inscribed temples with recipes and images depicting the preparation of oil-based scents. In Ancient Egypt, perfume was associated with the gods and, being expensive, was the preserve of the wealthy elite. The materials were hard to come by, and mounting an expedition to source sweet-smelling ingredients was a major and pricey undertaking. Egypt's status as a leading innovator of perfume is demonstrated by reports that when Julius Caesar took control of the country, he marked his triumphant return to Rome by tossing bottles of fragrance into the cheering crowds.

As trade routes opened up and economic power shifted, the use of perfume followed suit, traveling from Arabia to Greece and then the rest of Europe. In Rome, Emperor Nero, not known for scrimping on entertainment, used more frankincense at one wedding than could be produced in Arabia in a year. He also held banquets at which doves fluttered above the heads of guests on wings dipped in fragrant oils.

Creators of the Perfume Industry

Catherine de' Medici, a scion of the Italian banking family, is probably single-handedly responsible for the later French domination of the world of perfume. When Catherine married King Henry II of France in 1533, she insisted that he bring Italian perfumers to France and establish a French perfume industry. Centuries

---

Not to be Sniffed At

Antique and rare edition scent bottles were often made from cut glass and incorporated precious metals. Highly collectible and sought after, they frequently achieve high prices at auction. ❧

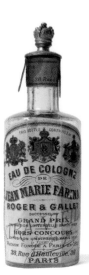
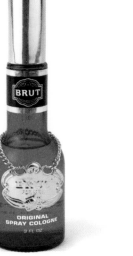
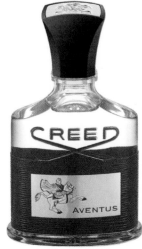

later, in the nineteenth century, this established industry saw an extraordinary blossoming. Paul Parquet has been described as "the greatest perfumer of his time" by none other than Ernest Beaux, the Franco-Russian perfumer who created Chanel No. 5. Parquet is recognized as the father of modern perfumery, chiefly through his championing of synthetics—aroma chemicals—in ground-breaking fragrances such as Fougère Royale by Houbigant, the perfume company of which Parquet was joint owner. In this, the first instance of an aroma chemical being employed in a perfume, he used a synthesized version of coumarin—a minute crystal found on the surface of the tonka bean. But instead of the labor-intensive work of scraping the bean's surface, the crystal was created in the lab using the new science of organic chemistry. It was 1882, and suddenly perfume could be produced far more cheaply, making it accessible to the masses instead of just a fragrant elite. Parquet suffered for his

innovation and was shunned by his fellow perfumers, who were affronted by his scientific dabblings, and the Church accused him of blasphemy for daring to tinker with God's creations. His work led, however, to the most exciting era for perfume and perfumers, a period lasting probably until about 1930.

Men's Fragrances

Men have been wearing fragrance since it was first invented. Ancient rulers—pharaohs, emperors, and kings—were anointed with oils, usually as part of a sacred ritual, and their clothing was soaked in scent. The rest of the populace was rather more unsavory, with the pungent aromas associated with lack of hygiene being reason enough to waft something more appealing under one's superior nose.

Napoléon Bonaparte was one such fellow famed for his love of scent. He is reported to have gone through four quarts of eau de Cologne a week, and Houbigant shipped their fragrances to the front line during the Napoleonic Wars. If you were going to die in battle you might as well be smelling your best.

By the 1970s, men's fragrances were becoming universally popular, creating an enthusiastic market for men's toiletries that has flourished ever since.

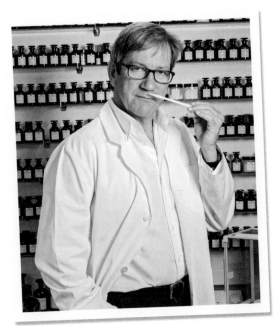

Scentimental Memories
Master perfumer John Stephen and his discerning nose (left). Ricki Hall's personal tribute (opposite).

CAPTAIN FAWCETT'S
BOOZE & BACCY BEARD OIL
CREATING A FRAGRANCE

Captain Fawcett is known for inventive collaborations with fellow gentlemen,
creating modern fragrances spiced with a personal story.

Captain Fawcett's Signature Series collaborations produce modern fragrances spiced with personal stories. When model and man-about-town Ricki Hall discussed creating a perfume based on his distinctive beard oil, it was clear this was a job for master perfumer John Stephen. A chartered chemist and one of only six independent perfumers in the U.K., John is the expert "nose" behind many fine fragrances, commissioned by top international perfume houses, and has produced two perfumes for the queen and fragrances for other members of the royal family.

Ricki's brief was clear. He wanted an intense male scent that reminded him of his late dad when he came home from the pub when Ricki was just a nipper. A man becomes deeply associated with the fragrance he wears, and the warmth of 1980s favorite Old Spice mixed with tobacco and beer was an emotional evocation of Ricki's boyhood and the men that era represented. Ricki said, "I was thinking about what men were like when I was a kid, strong blokes who didn't apologize for being masculine. I wanted to

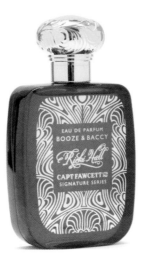

bring that back—the smell of being an adult in the '70s and '80s—booze, cigarettes, leather, aftershave, pubs—it's a bit of time travel."

Blending the right oils and ingredients to achieve the desired effect is where the perfumer becomes an alchemist. John explains, "When things blend or harmonize, something happens in the brain that puts these two things together, and they don't smell like two things any more. Perfect harmony is when you put two things together and you can't smell either of them—you smell a third thing. Our experience with fragrances is learned. It's a complex issue. When we experience smells, we can't take the sense of smell in isolation. Everything we experience is done through a multitude of senses, and then the brain puts that together and creates an experience that we understand life by."

A man becomes deeply associated with the fragrance he wears. Even in his absence, an unexpected hint of his familiar cologne resonates with all who know him. Although when asked what fragrance the master perfumer himself wears, John chuckles and answers "None!"

EXPLORING IDENTITY

The gentleman remains a recognizable figure through cultural change and shifting social mores, a constant across centuries and continents. This is precisely because fads and fashions, while they inspire and entertain, are not the essence of what it means to be a gentleman.

It is possible to identify where a gentleman stands in history by the mode of his dress, the style of his hair, the shape of his beard or mustache, and the tattoos he chooses to display or conceal. There are clues about the era in which he belongs in the scent of his fragrance, cut of his suit, angle of his hat, or color of his hosiery, and by whether he wears a watch, jewelery, or wig, but such historical markers are subject to continual change. These details are only the outward show of a complex inner life because joining the club of a true gentleman is not defined by accident of birth but by the expression of personality through habits and behavior.

Unconventional figures are blazing new trails though society. Men such as Eddie Izzard, marathon runner, comedian, actor, writer, and political campaigner, and Grayson Perry, artist and television presenter, exemplify the fluidity available to the modern gentleman or "transgentlemen." In fact, modern gentlemen's role models need not be men at all.

As old-school masculinity is re-evaluated and the lines between gender are increasingly blurred, style is changing to reflect the plurality of trans and non-binary gender experiences. The fashion world, despite its famed fickleness, is all-accepting in attitude, a conduit by which marginalized ideas might enter the mainstream, where taboos are broken and society reshaped.

In 2015 the London department store Selfridges sold clothing lines without stipulating whether they were intended for males or females, demonstrating the appeal of unisex aesthetics, and fashion houses increasingly use transgender models.

Much as the honored behavioral traits of gentlemen have been with us for centuries, ambiguity, androgyny, and cross-dressing are nothing new. From world folklore to the Elizabethan theater via women disguising themselves as men for careers as soldiers or pirates and the experimentation of Bloomsbury's literary set, the rules are always being challenged.

Life is moving at a frenetic pace. The modern gentleman is confident that his strength lies not in keeping up with relentless change but in accepting himself and being steadfast to his ideals. An egalitarian blend of the very best of his ancestors, he is treading his own path, gallant and thoughtful, respectful of tradition with an individual style always enlivened by a twist of dashing irreverence.

> "THE MODERN MAN SAVORS RITUALS OF GROOMING AND TAKES PLEASURE IN HIS DRESS NOT ONLY TO APPEAR AS A GENTLEMAN BUT PERCHANCE MORE IMPORTANTLY TO FEEL AND BEHAVE LIKE ONE."

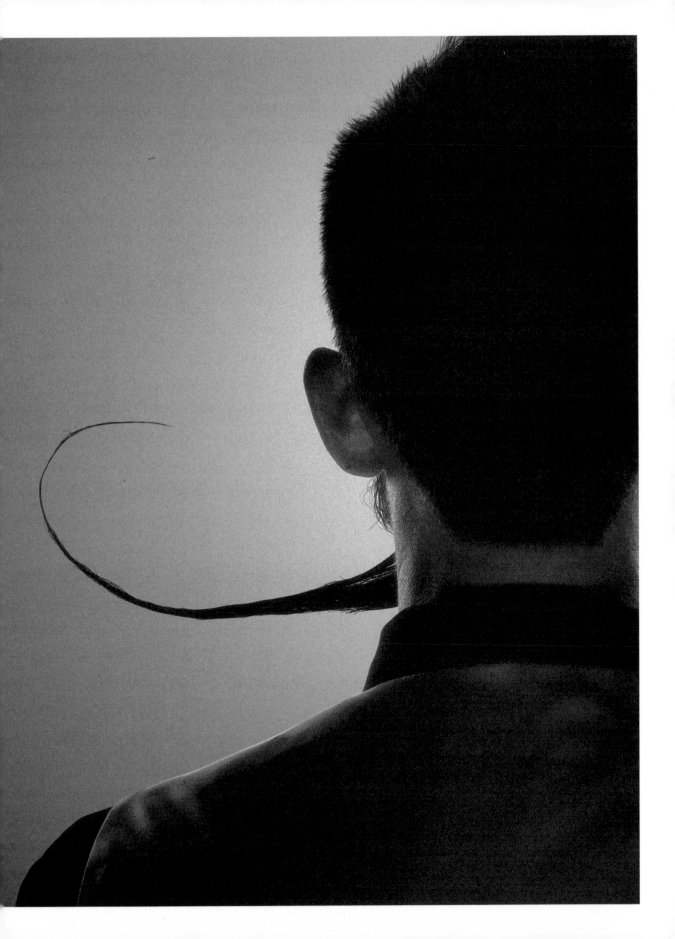

TOODLE PIP FROM THE CAPTAIN

AND SO MY dear companions of the page, the time has come for us to bid one another a most affectionate farewell. I hope, nay indeed trust, you have been tickled and transported by accompanying me on this jaunty excursion into the realm of the gentleman. We have seen that the way a man presents himself has an impact that both transcends time and makes its mark on history. When evidence is weighed in the balance, we find that the gentleman has always been here, manifest in all manner of society's many stations and spheres, from the center of the Earth to the very edge of the world and, as such, has always been "modern."

By reason of appearance alone, a perfectly quiet-living, even-tempered man might be scorned, celebrated, revered, feared, condemned, legislated against, and, most vexingly, taxed. For centuries, social commentators and wags from ancient Greek satirists to twenty-first-century comedians have sparred over the meaning of the face a man chooses to turn to his fellows. Take the enduring prevalence of the beard; is it an assertion of masculinity or a persistently recycled fashion? Perchance it is a rite of passage, a notion that every man should experiment with facial hair just because he can, and why not, by Jove! One must find ways to amuse oneself when the steam has been wiped from the bathroom mirror!

The codes of chivalry have shifted; I for one deal with the thoroughly modern dilemma of where to place a portable telephone by keeping it tucked away in one's pocket along with a compass, fob watch, and tin of expedition-strength mustache wax. Yet manners, simple acts of consideration and kindness, remain the very cornerstones of civilization, the principles which prevent us from falling into base savagery. One cannot emphasize strongly enough the quintessential necessity of being well groomed. Keeping up one's appearance, however individual and perchance eccentric it may seem to others, signifies that one takes care and preserves a regard for decorum that steps beyond the narrow boundary of the ego. The modern gentleman is the sum of his bearing, thoughts, and actions, the kind of chap who holds the door open not occasionally and not just for ladies, but always and for everyone.

Manners maketh man.

Most cordially & devotedly yours,

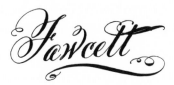

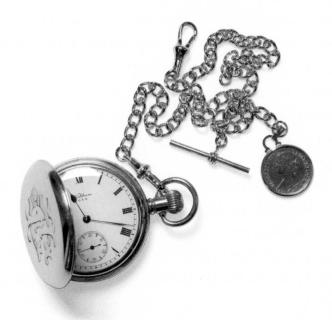

CREDITS & ACKNOWLEDGMENTS

The captain would like to take this opportunity to thank the photographers, artists, creative spirits, and intrepid travelers who were, in truth, the inspiration for this book.

(Key: a–above; b–below/bottom; c–center; f–far; l–left; r–right; t–top)

© **Tim Collins Photography** pp. 2 & 3 (The New York Barbershop, Rotterdam), 35, 42, 46, 75 (bl, bc, cr), 76, 77, 79, 85 (b), 87 (cl, tc, br), 96 & 97 (Schorem Barbers, Rotterdam), 98, 111, 112, 113, 118, 121, 130 & 131 (Schorem Barbers, Rotterdam), 156, 157, 165 (b). © **Quyen Dinh,** www.parlortattooprints. com @parlor tattoo_prints p. 4 © **Dominic Gregory** Photographer: Dominic Gregory at Zerovisuals.com (Savills Barbers, Sheffield) Suits by: John Lancaster – VS Mono pp. 8 & 9 © **Brock Elbank** pp. 13, 21 (b–l), 29 (c), 41, 47, 61 (c). © **Iain Crockart** pp. 7, 18, 36, 37, 38, 39, 40 (b), 44, 45, 49, 62, 63, 105, 171. © **Captain Fawcett Limited / Jacqui Small,** photography by Iain Crockart pp. 18 (beard token), 24 (b), 26 (t), 28, 31, 50 & 51 (Frank Rimer from Thy Barber: Shoreditch, London), 53 (t), 68, 69 70, 71, 72 (Banks Barbershop in Wisbech, Cambridgeshire), 73, 75 (br), 83 (t), 85 (t), 87 (cr), 90, 91, 92, 93, 94, 95, 132, 135, 138, 139, 140, 141, 142, 143, 144, 145, 152, 161, 162, 165 (t), 166, 167, 169, 170, 175. © **Cathleen Minton,** www.spritofthegreenman.co.uk p. 26 (tl) Thanks to Amy Rose at the

Barbershop Harmony Society p. 29 (tc) © **Joe and Jim at Heins Creative** p. 29 (lc) © **Vincent Kamp** p. 29 (bc) (Shaun Dixon, Cuts & Bruises) © **Project Barbatype (Scott Hilton and Bryan Wing)** p. 30 © **2007 Warner Bros. Entertainment Inc. and DreamWorks LLC. All Rights Reserved.** p. 34 © **Testoni Donato** p. 40 (t) © **Ben Gibson** p. 50 © **Matt Austin Images** p. 52 © **Susanne Jeurink-Timmer** p. 55(b) © **Ash Springle** p. 59 © **Dan Herrera** pp. 60 (tr) & 61 (cr) © **Greg Anderson Photography** pp. 60 (bl), 61 (tr, tl, br) & 173 © **Jeffrey Moustache** p. 60 (tl, tc, cr, br) © **Ed Reeve** pp. 64 & 65, 78 (bl), 80 (all Ludlow Blunt in Williamsburg, Brooklyn) **Congratulations to Photocrowd winners:** © **Fern Blacker** p. 75 (tr) © **Stefan Nielsen** p. 101, © **Nimit Nigam** p. 103, © **Nimai Chandra Ghosh** p. 104 (br), © **Navin Xavier** p. 104 (cl), © **Marco Tagliarino** p. 105 (tl), © **Shouvik Basak** p. 105 (tr), © **Willem Kuijpers** p. 104 (cr) & © **Paul Harley** p. 105 (bl) © **Rob Hammer** Photography p. 81,105 (cr, br) © **Kade Kut** Photography: Dan Davies, Two D Photography (Kade Kut, Image Barber) Makeup: Carrie-Anne Whitbread p. 86 © **Robin Bharaj** pp. 87 (c) & 125 © **Benedict Stenning** p. 87 (tl) © **Tariq**

Howes p. 87 (bl) (Fadez Barbershop Cardiff) © **Sonny McCartney** p. 87 (tr) © **Debby Besford Photography, 2016** pp. 88 & 89 © **Maciej Dakowicz** pp. 102 & 104 (tr, bl) © **Miguel Gutierrez, The Nomad Barber** pp. 104 (tl), 107, 108, 109 Thanks to Andrew Brewster from BarberEVO © **Johnny's Chop Shop** p. 114 © **Michael Barton** p. 115 © **Matt Spracklen** p. 117 © **Jelle Mollema Photography** p. 120 © **Dan Lord** p. 123

ACKNOWLEDGMENTS

Juliette Goggin and Abi Righton for their throughly modern recipes. Mike McCarthy for his simply splendid illustrations. Zacchary Falconer-Barfield, a perfect gentleman. The Bath Academy of Media Makeup. The loyal friends and colleagues who have offered advice, expertise, and innumerable pots of tea.

And last, but by certainly no means least, I salute the many barbers around the world who continue this noble profession. Long may you remain at the cutting edge!

Carry on …

The publisher would like to thank the following for their kind permission to reproduce their photographs:

Page 10: Magnum Photos / Philippe Halsman © Salvador Dali, Gala-Salvador Dali Foundation; Page 12: AF Fotografie; Page 14: Alamy / Peter Horree; Page 15 (t): Wellcome Library, London. Wellcome Images; Page 15 (b): Powerhouse Museum / Gift of the Estate of Raymond W Phillips, 2008; Page 16 (tl): Alamy / Uber Bilder; Page 16 (bl): Live Auctioneers / Ancient Resource, LLC; Page 16 (bcl): Alamy / age fotostock / J.D. Dallet; Page 16 (bcr): Alamy / World History Archive; Page 16 (br): Alamy / World History Archive; Page 17 (tr): The National Library of Medicine, U.S.A.; Page 17 (bl): Alamy / World History Archive; Page 17 (bcl): Alamy / Heritage Image Partnership Ltd / Werner Forman Archive; Page 17 (bcr): Alamy / Ian Dagnall; Page 17 (br): Alamy / Russell Hoban; Page 18 (bcl): Alamy / Classic Image; Page 18 (br): Alamy / State Hermitage Museum; Page 19: Alamy / War Archive; Page 20 (bl): NDSU, Institute for Regional Studies, Fargo (Folio 13.1); Page 20 (bcl): Alamy / Digital Image Library; Page 20 (bcr): Wellcome Library, London. Wellcome Images; Page 20

(br): Alamy / World History Archive; Page 21 (tr): AF Fotografie Page 21 (bl): Alamy / IanDagnall Computing; Page 21 (bcl): Alamy / Shawshots; Page 21 (bcr): Alamy / Mary Evans Picture Library; Page 23 (tl): Alamy / World Religions Photo Library; Page 23 (tcl): Alamy / Art Directors & TRIP / ArkReligion.com; Page 23 (tcr): Alamy / Rupert Sagar-Musgrave; Page 23 (tr): Alamy / robertharding / Donald Nausbaum; Page 23 (l): Alamy / imageBROKER / Tommy Seiter; Page 23 (cl): Rex / Shutterstock / Majority World; Page 23 (cr): Alamy / Victor Paul Borg; Page 23 (r): Alamy / Universal Images Group North America LLC; Page 24 (t): Bridgeman Images / National Army Museum, London / Colour: R Smithies; Page 25 (tr): AF Fotografie; Page 26 (br): Bridgeman Images / Archives Charmet / Private Collection; Page 27 (tr): Alamy / Prisma Archivo; Page 27 (b): AF Fotografie; Page 29 (tl): Getty / The LIFE Images Collection / Marvin Lichtner; Page 29 (tr): National Gallery of Art, Washington; Page 29 (r): Getty / Hulton-Deutsch Collection / Corbis; Page 29 (bc): Alamy / ITAR-TASS Photo Agency; Page 29 (br): Alamy / Picsstock; Page 31 (tl): Alamy / BFA; Page 31 (br): McDonald's; Page 32-33: Magnum Photos / Dennis Stock; Page 43:

Alamy / Everett Collection Inc; Page 54: Rex / Shutterstock / London News Pictures; Page 55 (tl): Alamy / pbpgalleries; Page 66: Bridgeman Images / The Advertising Archives / Private Collection; Page 74: AF Fotografie; Page 75 (tl): Wellcome Images / Science Museum, London; Page 75 (tc): AF Fotografie; Page 75 (l): AF Fotografie; Page 75 (c): 1st dibs; Page 82 (tl): Alamy / Claudine Klodien; Page 82 (b): Alamy / Paul Grover; Page 83 (br): Alamy / Ton Koene; Page 84: Adobe Stock / lynea; Page 134 (tl): Alamy / 503 collection; Page 136: Alamy / gameover; Page 137 (tl): Rex / Shutterstock / The Art Archive; Page 137 (tr): Wellcome Library, London. Wellcome Images; Page 137 (tc): Shutterstock / Gareth Howlett; Page 137 (cr): Wellcome Library, London. Wellcome Images; Page 137 (bl): Wellcome Library, London. Wellcome Images; Page 138 (br): Rex / Shutterstock / Granger; Page 144: AF Fotografie; Page 148: iStock / feedough; Page 153: Wellcome Library, London. Wellcome Images Page 154: AF Fotografie; Page 155: Wellcome Library, London. Wellcome Images; Page 160: Alamy / Granger Historical Picture Archive; Page 163: Magnum / Chris Steele-Perkins; Page 168: Alamy / Vintage Archives; Page 169 (bc): Alamy / Ian Dagnall; Page 169 (br): Creed.